HUMAN REPRODUCTIVE SYSTEM - ANATOMY, ROLES AND DISORDERS

INTRACYTOPLASMIC SPERM INJECTION (ICSI)

CLINICAL CONSIDERATIONS, OUTCOMES AND POTENTIAL HEALTH EFFECTS

HUMAN REPRODUCTIVE SYSTEM - ANATOMY, ROLES AND DISORDERS

Additional books and e-books in this series can be found on Nova's website under the Series tab.

HUMAN REPRODUCTIVE SYSTEM - ANATOMY, ROLES AND DISORDERS

INTRACYTOPLASMIC SPERM INJECTION (ICSI)

CLINICAL CONSIDERATIONS, OUTCOMES AND POTENTIAL HEALTH EFFECTS

MURID JAVED
EDITOR

nova
Medicine & Health
New York

NOTICE TO THE READER

The Publisher has taken reasonable care in the preparation of this book, but makes no expressed or implied warranty of any kind and assumes no responsibility for any errors or omissions. No liability is assumed for incidental or consequential damages in connection with or arising out of information contained in this book. The Publisher shall not be liable for any special, consequential, or exemplary damages resulting, in whole or in part, from the readers' use of, or reliance upon, this material. Any parts of this book based on government reports are so indicated and copyright is claimed for those parts to the extent applicable to compilations of such works.

Independent verification should be sought for any data, advice or recommendations contained in this book. In addition, no responsibility is assumed by the Publisher for any injury and/or damage to persons or property arising from any methods, products, instructions, ideas or otherwise contained in this publication.

This publication is designed to provide accurate and authoritative information with regard to the subject matter covered herein. It is sold with the clear understanding that the Publisher is not engaged in rendering legal or any other professional services. If legal or any other expert assistance is required, the services of a competent person should be sought. FROM A DECLARATION OF PARTICIPANTS JOINTLY ADOPTED BY A COMMITTEE OF THE AMERICAN BAR ASSOCIATION AND A COMMITTEE OF PUBLISHERS.

Additional color graphics may be available in the e-book version of this book.

Library of Congress Cataloging-in-Publication Data

ISBN: 978-1-53619-762-4

Published by Nova Science Publishers, Inc. † New York

CONTENTS

Preface

Increase in infertility around the globe is requiring the utilization of assisted reproductive technologies (ART). The basic ART include ovulation control and intrauterine insemination. The success rate is low and can't overcome infertility in many cases. Therefore, advanced ART techniques like *in-vitro fertilization* (IVF) and intracytoplasmic sperm injection (ICSI) are used. The first baby born by IVF was in 1978 and the ICSI was first used in human in 1992. Since then significant advances have been made in ART. The ICSI has enabled even those men who have rare sperm in their testes to father a biological child.

The ART enables those men and women to have a biological child who have deficiencies or defects in their reproductive system. The nature of these defects varies and could be congenital, acquired or genetic. The children born through ART are, therefore, considered at higher risk of carrying the defect found in parents. Many investigations have been carried out to compare incidence of the defects between children conceived naturally and conceived through ART. Additional technologies have been developed to ensure birth of a normal child. These include, pre-implantation genetic testing and non-invasive prenatal testing to verify the normality of the child.

This book covers different aspects of ART from basic to the advanced level. The first few chapters cover the introduction, scientific basis of sperm production and ways to enhance the fertilization. They identify the factors that affect success rate. One chapter focuses on a common condition in men, varicocele that deteriorates the sperm quality. It compares the outcome before and after the varicocele repair. A chapter addresses the abnormal fertilization and describes method to correct it. The effects of ICSI on the health of children are covered in Chapter 7 and finally the last chapter addresses the concern of passage of genetic defects from father to the offspring.

The authors of the chapters in this book are highly experienced and from different parts of the World. Many of them are directing very busy ART laboratories at leading infertility clinics in the United States of America, Canada and the Middle East. The knowledge in this book is expected to be useful for professionals, infertility patients and the common reader.

(Murid Javed, MSc (Hons), PhD)
Editor

In: Intracytoplasmic Sperm Injection (ICSI) ISBN: 978-1-53619-762-4
Editor: Murid Javed

Chapter 1

FACTORS AFFECTING INTRACYTOPLASMIC SPERM INJECTION FERTILIZATION RATE

Iman Halvaei[1], PhD and Navid Esfandiari[2,*], PhD, HCLD

[1]Department of Anatomical Sciences, Faculty of Medical Sciences, Tarbiat Modares University, Tehran, Iran
[2]Department of Obstetrics, Gynecology and Reproductive Sciences, University of Vermont Medical Center, Burlington, VT, US

ABSTRACT

This chapter explains factors affecting fertilization rate after intracytoplasmic sperm injection (ICSI). The poor fertilization may happen due to oocyte or sperm deficiencies or due to technical deficiency. Introduction of ICSI revolutionized the Assisted Reproductive Technology by increasing fertilization rate even in cases of severe male factor infertility. The common female factors affecting fertilization after ICSI include oocyte immaturity, low oocyte number, poor oocyte quality, abnormal oocytes, improper oocyte denuding and handling, and oocyte activation problem. The common male factors include all immotile sperm, extremely low sperm number, poor sperm motility, abnormal sperm morphology,

* Corresponding Author's E-mail: Navid.Esfandiari@uvmhealth.org.

high sperm DNA fragmentation, and absence of acrosome. Improper sperm processing, poor sperm selection and faulty ICSI technique are a few other factors affecting fertilization. In cases of failed fertilization after conventional IVF, rescue ICSI can be performed, however, there is no option after failed fertilization post ICSI.

Keywords: ICSI, rescue ICSI, total failed fertilization, oocyte morphology, testicular sperm

Introduction

A major disappointment that an infertile couple and the in vitro fertilization (IVF) team may face during an IVF cycle is unexpected total or partial fertilization failure. Several oocyte micromanipulation techniques have been developed to avoid fertilization failure following conventional insemination of oocytes including thinning or hatching the zona pellucida (ZP) and partial zona dissection (PZD). Subsequently, subzonal injection (SUZI) was introduced as a procedure where the sperm were injected beneath the zona in the perivitelline space. Intracytoplasmic sperm injection (ICSI), or the injection of a single spermatozoon into an oocyte under a microscope equipped with micromanipulator, was accidently introduced by Palermo in 1992 (Palermo, Joris et al. 1992). Introduction of ICSI is considered as one of the greatest achievements in the field of assisted reproductive technology (ART) helping infertile couples with severe male factor infertility and those who had experienced a failed fertilization from conventional IVF. The rate of fertilization following ICSI is estimated to be between 70-80% using ejaculated spermatozoa (Palermo, Neri et al. 2009).

Initially the only indication of ICSI was the male factor infertility but over the years it has been used for cases with non-ejaculated spermatozoa, previously cryopreserved gametes, *In vitro* matured eggs, and pre-implantation genetic testing (PGT).

ART is accounted for 1.5% of all infants born in the United States (Sunderam, Kissin et al. 2015) and according to International

Committee for Monitoring Assisted Reproductive Technology (ICMART) report, ICSI accounts for 66.5% of ART cycles worldwide (Adamson, de Mouzon et al. 2018). In some IVF programs, ICSI is used as method of fertilization for almost 100% of IVF cycles (Dyer, Chambers et al. 2016). The European Society of Human Reproduction and Embryology (ESHRE) has reported that 52.8% of 729,000 ART cycles performed in 2015 were ICSI cycles (De Geyter, Calhaz-Jorge et al. 2020). Several factors that can affect ICSI fertilization outcome are summarized in this chapter.

Oocyte Factors

Oocyte Maturity

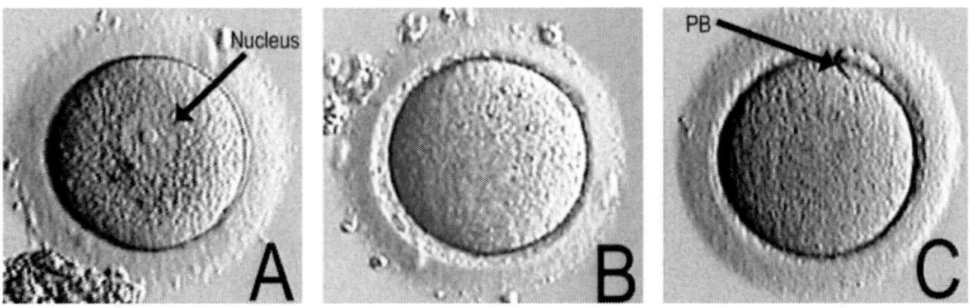

Figure 1. Oocyte development stages; (A) germinal vesicle (GV), At this stage the oocyte has 46 chromosomes and the nucleus is visible. (B) Metaphase I (MI), the nucleus dissolves but the first polar body is not extruded. (C) Metaphase II (MII), the first polar body is extruded.

Immature oocytes obtained following ovarian stimulation, including metaphase-I (MI) and germinal vesicle (GV) stage (Figure 1), have incomplete nuclear and cytoplasmic maturation and have low fertilization capability (Ebner, Yaman et al. 2001). ICSI is the method of choice to fertilize the *In vitro* matured oocytes (Haddad, Stewart et al. 2020), however the rate of fertilization is significantly lower in *In vitro* matured oocytes as compared to mature metaphase-II (MII) oocytes (De Vos, Van de Velde et al. 1999, Huang, Chang et al. 1999, Balakier, Sojecki et al. 2004, Strassburger, Friedler et al. 2004, De Vincentiis, De Martino et al. 2013, Shin, Cho et al. 2013). The number of immature oocytes in the cohort, or retrieved oocytes, affects the overall fertilization rate in mature oocytes. Recent studies have shown that increasing the number of immature oocytes decreases fertilization rate in sibling mature oocytes which indicates if the number of immature oocytes are high, sibling mature oocytes may also have suboptimal cytoplasmic maturation and low fertilization competence (Halvaei, Khalili et al. 2012, Parrella, Irani et al. 2019).

Oocyte Denudation

The cumulus and corona cells attached to ZP need to be removed prior to any micromanipulations using a combination of hyaluronidase and mechanical procedure (Figure 2).

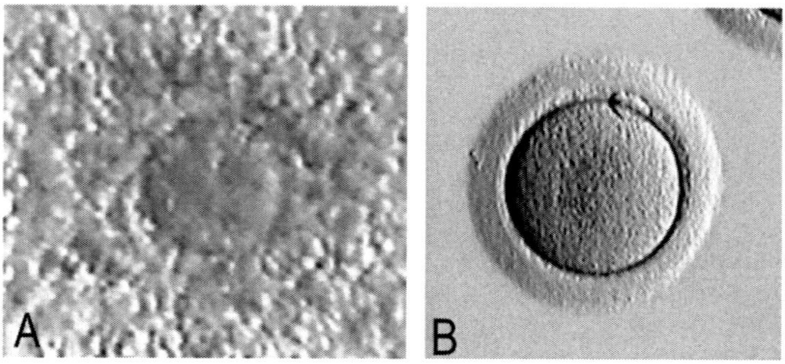

Figure 2. An oocyte retrieved from follicle, also called cumulus oocyte complex (A) and a denuded oocyte (B).

The concentration of the hyaluronidase utilized and the total time that oocytes are exposed are critical to the success of ICSI procedure. Van de Velde et al. showed that treating oocytes with 10 IU/mL hyaluronidase for a period of 30 sec is optimal for cumulus-corona cell removal (Van de Velde, De Vos et al. 1998). Aggressive oocyte manipulation during denudation, or use of a small size pipette for mechanical denudation results in higher rate of oocyte degeneration, and lowers ICSI fertilization rate (Nagy, Liu et al. 1995). Ebner et al. showed that partial oocyte denudation may improve cleavage stage embryo morphology as well as blastocyst formation, but renders the

ICSI procedure challenging and may increase the damage to oocytes as a result (Ebner, Moser et al. 2006).

Oocyte Morphology

Following cumulus-corona cell removal, the oocyte morphology is assessed under an inverted microscope. Different parts of the oocyte, including ZP, presence of polar body, and any cytoplasmic inclusions, can be accurately evaluated before microinjection. In general, oocyte dysmorphism is categorized into extra-cytoplasmic and cytoplasmic abnormalities. The etiology of morphological defects in oocyte is multifactorial and can be due to the ovarian stimulation protocol chosen and type of gonadotropin used (Haddad, Stewart et al. 2020). It is not uncommon for extra-cytoplasmic and cytoplasmic dysmorphisms to occur together in the same oocyte. The Figure 3 is showing common abnormalities observed in oocytes.

The role of oocyte morphology on ICSI fertilization rate has been a matter of several studies. A well designed systematic review of 50 studies in a period of 15 years could not draw a solid conclusion on the predictive potential of oocyte morphology in human IVF/ICSI outcome (Rienzi, Vajta et al. 2011). Some studies have shown that the oocyte can be fertilized regardless of oocyte morphological abnormalities (Sutter, Dozortsev et al. 1996, Balaban, Urman et al. 1998). Rienzi et al. evaluated 1,191 oocytes and found that cytoplasmic vacuoles, abnormal polar body, and large perivitelline space (PVS) could be related to decrease fertilization rate while other abnormalities such as fragmented polar body, abnormal ZP, abnormal oocyte shape, granular cytoplasm, central granulation, cluster of smooth endoplasmic reticulum (cSER), and presence of refractile bodies had no effects on fertilization rate (Rienzi, Ubaldi et al. 2008). It is suggested that some extra-cytoplasmic abnormalities such as first polar body morphology, large PVS and debris in PVS are signs of oocyte aging (ESHRE 2011). Palermo's group evaluated 129,412 oocytes over a 10-year period and showed that there was an inverse correlation between fertilization rate and proportion of oocytes with abnormal morphology in which the lowest fertilization rate was for oocytes having 75-100% dysmorphic features. Considering the effect of oocyte maturity, they included only the cycles with at least 70% mature oocytes and found again that fertilization rate was affected by the proportion of oocyte with dysmorphic features. However, this relationship was not significant when the cycles from female patients younger than 35 years were included. They showed that nuclear defects including fragmented polar body, large polar body, and two polar bodies significantly decreased fertilization rate compared to control group (74 vs 78.6%, respectively). They did not determine which sub-group of nuclear defects is responsible for worse outcome (O'Neill, Cheung et al. 2020).

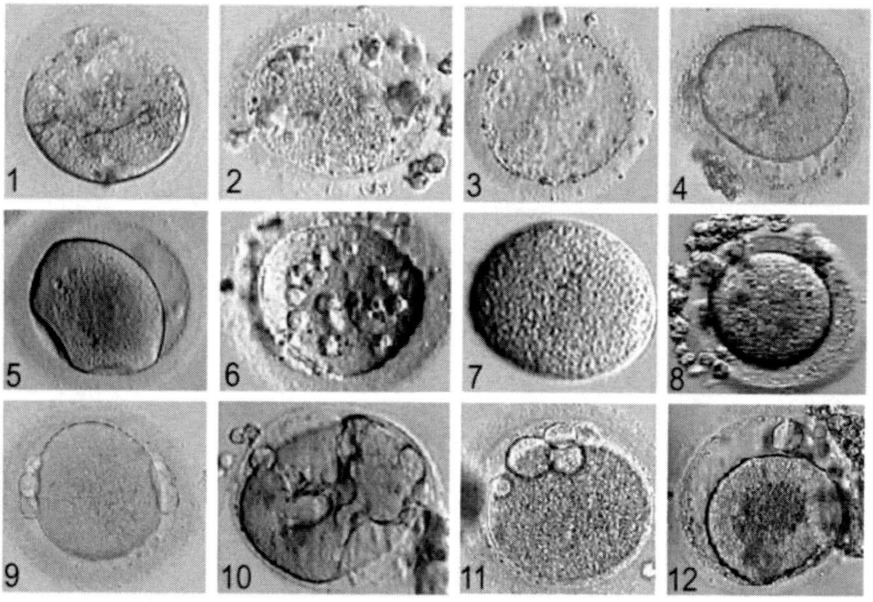

Figure 3. Common abnormalities found in oocytes after denudation; (1) Severely vacuolated degenerating oocyte, (2) Degenerated oocyte cytoplasm, (3) Empty zona pellucida, (4) Oocyte with a big vacuole, (5) Irregular cytoplasmic membrane and big perivitelline space, (6) An oocyte with multiple small vacuoles, (7) Zona-free oocyte, (8) Big perivitelline space, (9) An oocyte with fragmented polar bodies on opposite sides, (10) An oocyte with irregular cytoplasmic membrane, (11) An oocyte with multiple big polar body fragments, and (12) An oocyte with multiple defects (Central granularity, big perivitelline space and a big polar body).

Size and morphology of first polar body have been evaluated for its possible effect on fertilization outcome. It was shown that there was no relationship between polar body fragmentation and fertilization rate (Ebner, Moser et al. 2002, Ciotti, Notarangelo et al. 2004, De Santis, Cino et al. 2005, Navarro, de Araújo et al. 2009, Younis, Radin et al. 2009, Halvaei, Khalili et al. 2011). Verlinsky et al. evaluated embryos with different categories of polar body morphology and found no relationship between the shape of polar body and genetic competence of the oocytes (Verlinsky, Lerner et al. 2003). Interestingly and contrary to previous reports, researchers from Semmelweis University in Budapest found that the fertilization rate in oocytes with fragmented polar body was the highest in their study cohort (Fancsovits, Tóthné et al. 2006). Regarding the size of polar body, almost all reports are in favor of lower fertilization rate when the polar body is enlarged and some authors suggested that these oocytes are possibly aneuploid and should be discarded (Ebner, Yaman et al. 2000, Fancsovits, Tóthné et al. 2006, Navarro, de Araújo et al. 2009).

Effect of oocytes extra-cytoplasmic abnormalities on impaired fertilization following ICSI has been studied widely. Xia was the first who described the negative effects of a large PVS on the fertilization rate (Xia 1997). In regards to the presence of debris in the PVS, Hassan-Ali et al. found that the fertilization rate was similar between oocytes with >50% debris in the PVS and in oocytes with <50% debris in the PVS (Hassan-Ali, Hisham-Saleh et al. 1998). Zanetti et al. recently evaluated the impact of PVS abnormalities on ICSI outcomes using 9,752 oocytes obtained from 1,151 cycles and found that the presence of debris in the PVS, or a large PVS alone, or a combination of both anomalies in the oocytes may not affect fertilization rate (Zanetti, Braga et al. 2018). It has been shown that fertilization, embryo development, and successful pregnancy can be achieved from brown oocytes, characterized by dark granular appearance of the cytoplasm with or without inclusions and a thick ZP, at the same rate as embryos from morphologically normal oocytes (Esfandiari, Burjaq et al. 2006).

There are controversial reports on the relationship between the appearance of SER and fertilization rate following ICSI. It was shown that presence of SER has negative effects on the fertilization rate (Otsuki, Okada et al. 2004, Sá, Cunha et al. 2011). In a recent retrospective study, Massarotti et al. found SER aggregates in 2.8% of 12,436 metaphase II oocytes and found a significant reduction in the fertilization rate in the SER + oocytes (Massarotti, Stigliani et al. 2021). The refractile bodies are cytoplasmic inclusions and defined as dark incorporations within the cytoplasm and their impact on the fertilization rate of mature oocytes is a matter of debate. Khalili et al. showed negative effects of refractile bodies on fertilization rate, while Ebner et al. found that refractile bodies, or a dark cytoplasm/ZP, and an irregular shape of oocyte had no effect on fertilization rate (Ebner, Yaman et al. 2000, Khalili, Mojibian et al. 2005).

Vacuoles are among cytoplasmic inclusions that are found inside the oocyte with different sizes and numbers. Vacuoles are thought to be formed spontaneously, or following fusion of cytoplasmic vesicles (Van Blerkom 1990). The incidence of vacuoles in the oocyte can be up to 12.4%, with the mean diameter of vacuoles in the fertilized oocytes at 9.8 µm, and significantly larger (17.6 µm) in non-fertilized oocytes (Alikani, Palermo et al. 1995, Ebner, Moser et al. 2005). Ebner et al. reported that no fertilization was achieved in oocytes with vacuoles larger than 14 µm. They also concluded that the prognosis of the oocyte with multiple vacuoles was worse than the oocytes with a single vacuole. (Ebner, Moser et al. 2005). To improve the fertilization rate in oocytes with a varying number of vacuoles and/or SER, it is recommended that sperm should be deposited in cytoplasm away from these inclusions.

The effect of oocyte dysmorphism on fertilization rate in mild to severe male factor cases was studied by Ten et al. (2007) using 1,533 donor oocytes (Ten, Mendiola et al. 2007). They found that 94.5% of oocytes had at least one morphological abnormality. However, large PVS, debris in PVS, non-spherical shape of oocyte, abnormal ZP integrity, fragmented/irregular polar body, excessive cytoplasmic granularity, the presence of a vacuole, and dark cytoplasm had no effect on fertilization rate. It has been shown earlier that granular cytoplasm and centrally located granulation (slight or severe) does not affect fertilization outcome (Serhal, Ranieri et al. 1997, Kahraman, Yakın et al. 2000). Xia found that cytoplasmic inclusions are a determinant factor for fertilization rate. They also found that the rate of oocytes with cytoplasmic inclusions was significantly higher in female factor infertility and in women older than 35 years, and that large PVS without presence of cytoplasmic inclusion lowers the fertilization rate (Xia 1997). The effect of age on oocyte dysmorphism has been studied using 3,148 oocytes from 350 cycles and no relationship was found between age and oocyte dysmorphism (Rita de Cássia, Braga et al. 2010). The detrimental effects of cytoplasmic dysmorphism on impaired fertilization may be related to cytoskeletal changes and meiotic spindle functions where the second polar body should be extruded and pronuclei formed (Rita de Cássia, Braga et al. 2010). Wilding et al. evaluated oolema behavior, pattern of cytoplasmic granularity, and presence of vacuoles or inclusions on ICSI outcomes from 6,397 oocytes (822 patients) and found that absence of granularity, presence of both inclusions and vacuoles, and easy to break oolema resulted in the lowest fertilization rate (Wilding, Di Matteo et al. 2007).

Oocyte size and its mean diameter are proposed as predictors of fertilization, embryo quality, and blastocyst development. The oocyte is called giant when the diameter of an oocyte is larger than 200 μm. The giant oocytes are diploid mainly due to faulty mitotic division or fusion of two oogonia and they comprise less than 1% of retrieved oocytes (Balakier, Bouman et al. 2002, Ebner, Moser et al. 2006). It seems that large size of oocyte is not associated with decreased fertilization rate, but it is suggested these oocytes should be discarded due to their high aneuploidy rate (Rosenbusch, Schneider et al. 2002, Ebner, Moser et al. 2006).

Viscosity of oocyte cytoplasm is another feature that has been evaluated for possible effects on fertilization rate. Ebner et al. evaluated the oocyte viscosity by assessment of the formation of a funnel in the membrane after withdrawal of injecting needle and found that fertilization rate was not affected by viscosity of cytoplasm (Ebner, Moser et al. 2003). The combined morphological abnormality in comparison with single abnormality results in similar fertilization rate (Sutter, Dozortsev et al. 1996, Balaban, Urman et al. 1998, Loutradis, Drakakis et al. 1999). In a patient with history of failed intrauterine insemination (IUI) cycles undergoing an IVF cycle, Esfandiari et al. showed that oocytes with severe morphological abnormalities including irregular ZP, abnormal PVS, and cytoplasmic inclusions resulted in normal fertilization and a take home baby (Esfandiari, Ryan et al. 2005).

One of the most important factors that impacts oocyte quality is controlled ovarian hyperstimulation (Baart, Macklon et al. 2009), but its effects on fertilization rate is matter of debate. Imthurn et al. evaluated the effect of human menopausal gonadotrophin (HMG) and highly purified follicle stimulating hormone (FSH HP) on oocyte maturity and morphology. They found that the rate of oocyte maturity was higher in FSH HP group while the rate of dark cytoplasm was higher in HMG group. Nonetheless, fertilization rate was similar between the two groups (Imthurn, Macas et al. 1996). In a similar study, the effect of HMG and recombinant human FSH on oocyte quality was investigated and found that the rates of nuclear maturity and oocyte dysmorphism (extra- and cytoplasmic) were similar between two groups, and fertilization rate was also not significantly different (Rashidi, Sarvi et al. 2005).

Oocyte Activation

Oocyte activation is a key step among fundamental changes that happens during oocyte fertilization and is triggered following sperm-egg fusion (Horner and Wolfner 2008). Oocyte activation may not occur in 40-70% of unfertilized oocytes following ICSI mainly due to either sperm or oocyte defects (Yanagida 2004). Calcium (Ca^{++}) release inside the oocyte and Ca^{++} oscillations are key factors of oocyte activation following sperm entering the oocyte (Ramadan, Kashir et al. 2012). It was known that a sperm derived factor is released from the fertilizing sperm and can modulate Ca^{++} channels on the ER to release Ca^{++}. Both nuclear and cytoplasmic maturation are needed for the oocytes to respond to sperm factor. Following the entry of a sperm into ooplasm, mammalian zygote development is initiated by sperm-mediated Ca^{++} oscillations that remains until two pronuclei are formed (Jones 2005). Unlike conventional IVF, the increase in Ca^{++} starts immediately after the injection of spermatozoon which is due to artificial Ca^{++} influx from the surrounding injection medium (Tesarik, Mendoza et al. 2000) triggering essential alterations inside the oocytes, both nuclear and cytoplasmic, and inducing a successful fertilization. The physiological stimulus that precedes the cytosolic Ca^{++} oscillations is a testis-specific phospholipase C (PLC) isoform known as PLC-zeta (PLCzeta). Inhibition of PLC can block the initiation of Ca^{++} oscillations leading to failed fertilization (Yoon, Eum et al. 2012).

Artificial oocyte activation (AOA) aims to induce Ca^{++} oscillations inside the oocyte similar to the process in normal physiology. AOA can be done through chemical, mechanical, and electrical methods to overcome oocyte activation failure (Rubino, Viganò et al. 2016). Some chemicals including inomycin, calcimycin, or strontium have been used to overcome fertilization failure (Simopoulou, Giannelou et al. 2016). The first successful oocyte activation was obtained from using Ca^{++} ionophore in a globozoospermic patient (Battaglia, Koehler et al. 1997). Mechanical approach for oocyte activation is a modified ICSI technique where the cytoplasm of oocyte is vigorously aspirated. This technique is thought to have a similar effect of Ca^{++} ionophore (Tesarik and Sousa 1995). Egashira et al. reported a 100% fertilization rate following combination of ICSI and laser-assisted oocyte activation (Egashira, Murakami et al. 2009). Aydinuraz et al. in a prospective randomized sibling study found that using Ca^{++} ionophore immediately after intracytoplasmic morphologically selected sperm injection (IMSI) improved fertilization rate compared to the control group (82.5 vs 73.2%, respectively) (Aydinuraz, Dirican et al. 2016). Some studies using AOA in patients with previous conventional ICSI failure showed a significantly higher fertilization rate (Baltaci, Ayvaz et al. 2010, Vanden Meerschaut, Nikiforaki et al. 2012). A recent meta-analysis showed these studies might suffer from a high level bias risk and that there is insufficient evidence available from the included randomized controlled trials to justify the efficacy and safety of ICSI-AOA for couples with previous fertilization failure (Sfontouris, Nastri et al. 2015).

RESCUE ICSI AND *IN VITRO* OOCYTE AGING

Total fertilization failure is not very common in IVF, but it carries a high emotional and financial burden for the infertile couple. To attempt rescue of a cycle in the case of failed fertilization, re-insemination of unfertilized oocytes is performed with conventional insemination, or ICSI. It has been shown that in 1-day-old oocytes, the ZP hardens and the premature release of cortical granules further limits sperm–zona binding, therefore conventional re-insemination might not be an effective modality to rescue unfertilized eggs. It might be beneficial to inject sperm into the oocyte (rescue ICSI) to avoid cycle cancellation in patients with failed fertilization. Rescue ICSI should be performed as early as possible to avoid further aging of oocytes in culture (Esfandiari, Claessens et al. 2008). Morton et al. evaluated the outcomes of 439 oocytes from 54 cycles with complete fertilization failure and reported fertilization rate of 44% with high rate of aneuploidy in derived embryos (Morton, Yoder et al. 1997).

Oocyte Incubation Prior to ICSI

In stimulated cycles, nuclear and cytoplasmic maturation in oocytes might be asynchronized (Sundström and Nilsson 1988). Asynchrony between nuclear and cytoplasmic maturation can cause total or partial failed fertilization. Incubation of oocytes, with or without cumulus cells, before ICSI is beneficial for cytoplasmic maturation. There is no general agreement on the optimal timing of ICSI, with reports suggesting a wide range of duration of oocyte pre-incubation between 2.5 h to 12 h to improve fertilization rate (Rienzi, Ubaldi et al. 1998, Ho, Chen et al. 2003, Falcone, Gambera et al. 2008). An increased fertilization rate has been reported with a longer time interval between human chorionic gonadotropin (hCG) administration and oocyte retrieval (>36 h vs <36 h) (Garor, Shufaro et al. 2015), and 37 h vs 41 h in another study (Dozortsev, Nagy et al. 2004).

The effect of time interval between oocyte retrieval and denudation on ICSI fertilization outcome has also been a well-debated topic. A retrospective analysis of 1,378 ICSI cycles by Carvalho et al., has shown that fertilization rate was significantly higher when this interval was ≥4 h as compared to <3 h. In addition they evaluated the effect of time interval between oocyte retrieval and ICSI and found that fertilization rate was comparable between different groups (<5 h, 5-6 h, and >6 h) (Carvalho, Leal et al. 2020). However, not all investigators have found this association and there are also some conflicting data regarding the optimum time from oocyte retrieval to cytoplasmic injection. (Van de Velde, De Vos et al. 1998, Patrat, Kaffel et al. 2012, Garor, Shufaro et al. 2015). In an early study, it was shown that time between oocyte retrieval to ICSI (1 – 11 h) does not affect fertilization rate (Yanagida, Yazawa et al. 1998). Jacobs et al. reported the same findings for 0.5-8 h pre-incubation time between oocyte retrieval and injection (Jacobs, Stolwijk et al. 2001). While fertilization rate may not be influenced by different incubation time periods, pre-incubation of cumulus-oocyte-complex may increase the number of mature oocytes available for injection (Ho, Chen et al. 2003). In addition, it is shown that meiotic spindle appearance is time-dependent and most oocytes had distinct spindles 39-40.5 h post hCG injection, and this time interval is suggested as an optimum interval between hCG injection and ICSI (Kilani, Cooke et al. 2011). Given many factors affecting ICSI fertilization outcome, each IVF clinic needs to determine the optimum timing for ICSI procedure internally.

Sperm Factors

Sperm Count, Motility and Viability

Sperm count and motility are important factors affecting fertilization rate in ICSI cycles. Several studies have reported a reduced fertilization rate following ICSI in patients with sperm concentration <1 M/mL compared to those with sperm concentration ≥15 M/mL (Bartolacci, Pagliardini et al. 2018). In addition, in patients with sperm concentration <1 M/mL, fertilization rate is significantly decreased when the sperm motility is <10% as compared to those with ≥32%. Presence of multiple abnormal sperm characteristics negatively affects fertilization rate (Bartolacci, Pagliardini et al. 2018). Necrozoospermia, the presence of only nonviable sperm in ejaculate, and severe asthenozoospermia are associated with very low fertilization following ICSI (Ortega, Verheyen et al. 2011). The low fertilization rate in patients with severe asthenozoospermia, seems to be due to the injection of a non-viable spermatozoa instead of viable ones. It appears that the fertilization failure is due to the inability of a dead spermatozoa to activate the oocyte (Ahmadi and Ng 1999, Yazawa, Yanagida et al. 2009). In these patients, sperm retrieval from the testis (through aspiration or biopsy) might yield some viable and motile sperm cells (Ortega, Verheyen et al. 2011).

To improve motility, sperm have been treated with different compounds including theophylline and pentoxifylline (PTX). The PTX is a nonselective phosphodiesterase inhibitor and raises the intracellular level of cAMP in sperm cells, which in turn increases sperm motility (Buffone, Wertheimer et al. 2014). Using PTX to improve motility of frozen-thawed immotile testicular sperm resulted in an increased fertilization rate, and lowered the duration of the ICSI procedure as it facilitated the detection of viable spermatozoa (Kovačič, Vlaisavljević et al. 2006). The hypo-osmotic swelling test (HOST) is another method utilized during ICSI to differentiate viable sperm. In this test, spermatozoa are exposed to a hypo-osmotic solution and the sperm viable tails swell. Swelling patterns are categorized from 'a' to 'g' (Organization 2010). 'A'-spermatozoa are considered dead, while 'b' to 'g'-spermatozoa are alive and can be selected for ICSI (Soares, Glina et al. 2003). There are conflicting results regarding the use of HOST during ICSI for improving fertilization rate (Casper, Meriano et al. 1996, El-Nour, Al Mayman et al. 2001). However, the usefulness of HOST on successful fertilization in patients with Kartagener's syndrome has been reported in several case reports (Westlander, Barry et al. 2003, Kordus, Price et al. 2008). In a study comparing PTX and HOST for viability to identify viable testicular sperm with a functional intact membrane, it was shown that fertilization rate was significantly higher by sperm treated with PTX as compared to those sperm selected using HOST (62.05% vs. 41.07%, respectively) (Mangoli, Mangoli et al. 2011).

Myoinositol is a stereoisomer of inositol that affects intracellular concentration of Ca^{++}. It was shown that incubation of oligoastheno-teratospermic samples with myoinositol improved sperm motility and resulted in a higher fertilization rate following ICSI (Rubino, Palini et al. 2015). In addition to chemical compounds, the sperm tail flexibility test during sperm selection for ICSI helps the embryologist to select viable sperm. In this procedure, the injection needle touches and pushes the sperm tail in which the viable sperm has flexible tail where the movement of tail and head is independent to each other (Soares, Glina et al. 2003). Although this technique is easy and cost-effective, utilization requires experience and skillset.

Another method for detection of viable immotile sperm is the application of laser. In this technique, a coiled sperm tail following single laser shot is an indication of sperm viability. It seems laser-assisted sperm selection improves fertilization rate in absolute asthenozoospermia and testicular spermatozoa (Nordhoff, Schüring et al. 2013). Atkan et al. showed that compared to the selection of sperm through HOST, the fertilization rate was significantly higher when the laser was used for sperm selection in asthenozoospermia (64.2 versus 46.5%, respectively) (Aktan, Montag et al. 2004).

Sperm Morphology

There is little evidence for an association between sperm morphology and ICSI fertilization outcome. French et al. did not find any relationship between sperm morphology and fertilization rate (French, Sabanegh Jr et al. 2010). Globozoospermia is a monomorphic teratozoospermia where only round head sperm are present in the ejaculate and this abnormality accounts for <0.1% of male infertility (Rubino, Palini et al. 2015). These round-head sperm lack acrosome, have abnormal nuclear membrane, and midpiece anomalies (Singh 1992). Globozoospermic men are infertile and conventional IVF is ineffective because of lack of acrosome. The ICSI is method of choice for treatment of globozoospermic men. In addition, globozoospermia is associated with a high level of sperm DNA fragmentation, and aneuploidy (Perrin, Coat et al. 2013). It was found that PLCzeta is reduced, or absent, in globozoospermia and low fertilization in these patients is mainly due to the impaired oocyte activation. As mentioned earlier, AOA has been used to overcome fertilization failure in globozoospermic patients (Kuentz, Vanden Meerschaut et al. 2013).

Sperm DNA

The importance of sperm DNA fragmentation to IVF outcomes has been well debated. Although DNA fragmentation has been associated with decreased rate of successful pregnancy, the current literature on the effects of DNA fragmentation on fertilization rate following ICSI are conflicting. Several studies have found an inverse relationship between sperm DNA fragmentation and fertilization rate (Benchaib, Braun et al. 2003). In contrast, there is a body of evidence that rules out the negative effect of DNA fragmentation index (DFI) on ICSI fertilization outcome (Benchaib, Braun et al. 2003, Henkel, Kierspel et al. 2003, Huang, Lin et al. 2005, Benchaib, Lornage et al. 2007, Caglar, Köster et al. 2007, Simon, Brunborg et al. 2010, Speyer, Pizzey et al. 2010, Esbert, Pacheco et al. 2011, Pregl Breznik, Kovačič et al. 2013, Al Omrani, Al Eisa et al. 2018). Palermo et al. found no significant difference between two groups of patients with low DFI (<30%) and high DFI (>30%) (Palermo, Neri et al. 2014). Similarly, a lack of relationship between fertilization rate and single- and or double-stranded DNA damage was shown in a recent study (Casanovas, Ribas-Maynou et al. 2019). Alvarez et al. and Sun et al. evaluated fertilization rate between two groups with DFI >15% and <15% (by TUNEL assay) and DFI <30 and ≥30% (by SCD assay), respectively, and showed similar fertilization rate in both groups (Alvarez Sedó, Bilinski et al. 2017, Sun, Zhang et al. 2018).

Several researchers investigated the reproductive outcome in oligozoospermic men with high sperm DNA fragmentation undergoing ICSI with ejaculated and testicular sperm and reported that sperm DFI was significantly lower in testicular sperm when compared to ejaculated counterparts. They concluded that in selected oligozoospermic patients or those with non-obstructive azoospermia with high DFI, ICSI using testicular sperm might be beneficial (Greco, Scarselli et al. 2005, Esteves, Sánchez-Martín et al. 2015). However, investigating DNA fragmentation of testicular sperm has proved to be challenging. One study however, reported that sperm DNA fragmentation negatively affects fertilization rate mainly in IVF cycles and ICSI might be a preferred method of fertilization in cases with high DFI (Oleszczuk, Giwercman et al. 2016).

Sperm Source

Several studies have reported that the source of sperm (from ejaculate, epididymis, or testis) may affect ICSI fertilization rates. One study on unselected patients found that the rate of fertilization was significantly higher with ejaculated spermatozoa compared to epididymal and testicular samples, despite increased maternal age in this group, while ICSI using testicular sperm resulted in the lowest fertilization rate even in couples with young maternal age (Palermo, Neri et al. 2015). In another study, the fertilization rate following ICSI using ejaculated sperm and sperm obtained from the epididymal aspiration were similar but significantly higher compared with testicular sperm (60.6, 57.2 and 42.6%, respectively (Palermo, O'Neill et al. 2017). While no beneficial effects of testicular sperm for increasing fertilization rate in patients with cryptozoopermia were found in one meta-analysis (Abhyankar, Kathrins et al. 2016), Kang and his colleagues showed in their meta-analysis that testicular sperm is superior to ejaculated sperm for ICSI in males with cryptozoospermia (Kang, Hsiao et al. 2018). In patients with severe and complete asthenozoospermia, testicular aspirated sperm does not seem to improve fertilization rates following ICSI (Al-Malki, Alrabeeah et al. 2017). A meta-analysis on ICSI fertilization outcomes using fresh and frozen-thawed testicular sperm in non-obstructive azoospermia found that the fertilization rate was similar between fresh versus cryopreserved-thawed testicular sperm (Ohlander, Hotaling et al. 2014). The lack of consistent findings on ICSI outcomes using ejaculated or testicular sperm is likely in part due to small sample sizes, lack of a proper control group, and differing methods of DNA fragmentation testing.

Sperm Selection

The presence of any damage in sperm genome results in fertilization failure, poor quality embryos, an increase in miscarriage rate or a reduction in pregnancy and delivery rates. Therefore selecting sperm with intact DNA for ICSI is important. Several methods, including annexin V–magnetic activated cell sorting (MACS), zeta potential, electrophoretic separation, and hyaluronan binding assay (HBA) for selecting sperm with intact DNA have been recently described. Kheirollahi-Kouhestani et al. reported an increased fertilization rate following sperm selection by zeta potential (Kheirollahi-Kouhestani, Razavi et al. 2009). However, the reports on improved fertilization rates using sperm selected by annexin V-MACS are conflicting (Dirican, Isik et al. 2008, Dirican, Özgün et al. 2008, Sheikhi, Jalali et al. 2013). Other studies have found no positive effect of HBA sperm selection on fertilization rates (Nasr-Esfahani, Razavi et al. 2008, Parmegiani, Cognigni et al. 2010, Parmegiani, Cognigni et al. 2010). Similarly, a meta-analysis that evaluated seven studies on more than 9,700 injected oocytes found that the range of fertilization rate varied from 65 to 93% and from 65 to 87% in the hyaluronic acid (HA) and control groups respectively, and concluded that ICSI using sperm selected by HA does not improve fertilization rates (RR: 1.02, 95% CI: 0.99-1.06) (Beck-Fruchter, Shalev et al. 2016). It is suggested that an experienced and well-trained embryologist might be able to select sperm as good as HA-assisted sperm selection in terms of DNA integrity (Huang, Lee et al. 2015). This claim, however, needs to be validated by properly designed studies. Polarized microscopy, sperm head birefringence, polscope, and microfluidics have been used for sperm selection with varying results (Gianaroli, Magli et al. 2010, Ghosh, Chattopadhyay et al. 2012, Vermey, Chapman et al. 2015, Parrella, Keating et al. 2019).

METHODS OF SPERM PREPARATION

Swim-up and density gradient centrifugation are the most widely used techniques for sperm processing. Both methods yield high quality motile spermatozoa (Kim, Kim et al. 2015). It is suggested that if both techniques are combined, better quality sperm in terms of motility and morphology are selected and higher fertilization rates could be obtained especially when the sperm motility is under 50% (Simopoulou, Gkoles et al. 2016).

Intracytoplasmic Morphologically Selected Sperm Injection (IMSI)

During the ICSI procedure, the embryologist identifies morphologically normal sperm to directly inject into the oocyte. In a routine embryology practice, a magnification of ×400 enables the embryologist to identify any major sperm morphological defect. However, motile sperm organelle morphology examination (MSOME) provides the evaluation of sperm under much higher magnification at ×6000 to assess nuclear status and especially for presence of any vacuoles (Setti, Braga et al. 2013). The IMSI, therefore, is a modified ICSI technique using sperm that are selected under high magnification. The IMSI has been recommended for patients with repeated ICSI failure and those with sperm high DNA fragmentation (Setti, Braga et al. 2013).

There are some conflicting data regarding fertilization outcomes following IMSI. In a five-year prospective study in patients with failed ICSI or severe sperm head abnormality, it was found that fertilization rates following IMSI were higher compared to ICSI (80.6 versus 77.7%, respectively) (Cassuto, Hazout et al. 2014). Other studies have reported increased fertilization rates following IMSI compared to ICSI, with one study finding a higher fertilization rate in patient with oligoasthenoteratozoospermia with motile sperm count below 0.1×10^6 mL^{-1}, in patients with teratozoospermia (Goswami, Sharma et al. 2018), and in cycles where maternal age is older than 30 (Cassuto, Bouret et al. 2009). The latter study is in contrast to the Setti et al. study where the authors did not find an improvement in fertilization rates following IMSI in advanced maternal age (Setti, Figueira et al. 2013). Balaban et al. also found no improvement in fertilization rates in comparison with ICSI cycles in an unselected population of infertile patients (Balaban, Yakin et al. 2011) which is in line with findings of Marci et al. (Marci, Murisier et al. 2013). The IMSI did not improve fertilization rates in patients with poor quality semen samples (Knez, Zorn et al. 2011), patients with sperm DNA fragmentation >30% (Braga, Setti et al. 2011), patients with repeated implantation failure (Oliveira, Cavagna et al. 2011), and those with repeated IVF-ICSI failure (Shalom-Paz, Anabusi et al. 2015). In addition, in a randomized sibling oocyte study in patients with male factor undergoing ICSI, no significant difference for fertilization rates between ICSI and IMSI groups was found (De Vos, Van de Velde et al. 2013). Recently, Gaspard et al. conducted a retrospective two-center analysis of 573 ICSI and 275 IMSI cycles and found that fertilization rates were similar between ICSI and IMSI groups in patients with mild to severe oligo-, astheno-, and/or teratozo-ospermia, history of previous implantation failures after ICSI, decreased blastocyst development in previous cycles, repeated spontaneous abortions, low oocyte counts, or advanced maternal age (Gaspard, Vanderzwalmen et al. 2018). It seems that conflicting results on IMSI effectiveness come mainly from different inclusions criteria, ovarian stimulation protocol, sperm and oocyte quality, as well as ICSI inter-operator variability.

ICSI Technique

In order to reduce physical and chemical stress to the oocytes, ICSI procedure should be done as quickly as possible and injected oocytes returned to the incubator. During the ICSI procedure a morphologically normal sperm cell is selected and immobilized. Using a fine glass pipette the oocyte cytoplasmic membrane is breached and a single sperm is deposited inside the cytoplasm. Normal fertilization rate following the ICSI procedure is around 70%, while a small portion of oocytes might be damaged by the procedure. Oocyte damage following ICSI is mainly due to the poor quality of the oocyte, the quality and size of injecting needle, or the expertise of the embryologist performing ICSI. There are some conflicting reports regarding the effect of an embryologist's skillset on ICSI fertilization rates. In one study, Dumoulin et al. did not find any differences in fertilization rates between four ICSI operators (Dumoulin, Coonen et al. 2001), while in other studies, it was shown that ICSI operators may affect fertilization rate (Shen, Khabani et al. 2003, McCulloh, Goorbarry et al. 2011).

A faulty ICSI technique including excessive cytoplasmic manipulation, damaging or perforating the oolema on the opposite side of injection by deep insertion of pipette, injecting a large volume of fluid together with sperm, and large or blunt injection pipettes may increase oocyte degeneration rate after ICSI and decrease overall fertilization rate (Rubino, Viganò et al. 2016). During ICSI, a small volume of cytoplasm is aspirated inside the pipette to ensure membrane break and to mechanically activate the oocyte, however, Mansour et al. have shown that the oocyte can be fertilized without cytoplasmic aspiration during the ICSI procedure (Mansour, Aboulghar et al. 1996).

Usually meiotic spindle remains near the first polar body, and in order to reduce the risk of damaging the spindles, the embryologist positions the first polar body either at 6 or 12 o'clock and inserts the ICSI pipette at 3 o'clock (Dumoulin, Coonen et al. 2001). Earlier studies did not show any differences in fertilization rates with the polar body positioned at 6 or 12 o'clock (Nagy, Liu et al. 1995, Stoddart and Fleming 2000), however, Van der Westerlaken et al. reported an improved fertilization rate when the polar body was at 6 o'clock (Van der Westerlaken, Helmerhorst et al. 1999). In one study, it was shown that positioning the polar body at 11 o'clock is in favor of increased fertilization rate (Anifandis, Dafopoulos et al. 2010). Several other studies have also shown that visualization of the meiotic spindle using a polscope before ICSI increases the rate of fertilization (Wang, Meng et al. 2001, Wang, Meng et al. 2001, Moon, Hyun et al. 2003). Maintaining the optimum temperature during ICSI is also important as keeping oocytes at room temperature before ICSI may result in irreversible disruption of the meiotic spindle (Aman and Parks 1994).

Sperm immobilization prevents oocyte structural damage from sperm motility after deposition of the motile sperm inside the oocyte, and helps oocyte activation. Sperm are immobilized when their tails are scored by the injection pipette against the micromanipulation dish or by laser beam (Montag, Rink et al. 2000). Polyvinylpyrrolidone (PVP) solution is mostly used to facilitate sperm immobilization for ICSI procedure. Sperm immobilization induces permeability of the sperm plasma membrane and as mentioned earlier the release of sperm cytosolic factors into the oocyte and Ca^{++} oscillations are required for oocyte activation.

ICSI Pipette

The ICSI technique requires micro-tools including injection and holding pipettes (or needles). The injection pipette should be sharp and beveled. The inner diameter of the needle should be wide enough to enable the sperm entry into the pipette. The outer diameter of the needle also should not be too large to make a large hole in the cytoplasmic membrane and cause damage to the oocyte. A smaller inner diameter of the ICSI pipette leads to a reduced amount of PVP or culture media delivered to the oocyte, reduced mechanical pressure to the oocyte, and also minimizes the amount of aspirated cytoplasm into the pipette, resulting in a reduced rate of oocyte degeneration (Yavas, Roberge et al. 2001).

References

[1] Abhyankar, N., M. Kathrins and C. Niederberger (2016). "Use of testicular versus ejaculated sperm for intracytoplasmic sperm injection among men with cryptozoospermia: a meta-analysis." *Fertility and sterility* 105(6): 1469-1475. e1461.

[2] Adamson, G. D., J. de Mouzon, G. M. Chambers, F. Zegers-Hochschild, R. Mansour, O. Ishihara, M. Banker and S. Dyer (2018). "International Committee for Monitoring Assisted Reproductive Technology: world report on assisted reproductive technology, 2011." *Fertility and sterility* 110(6): 1067-1080.

[3] Ahmadi, A. and S. C. Ng (1999). "Fertilizing ability of DNA-damaged spermatozoa." *Journal of experimental zoology* 284(6): 696-704.

[4] Aktan, T., M. Montag, S. Duman, H. Gorkemli, K. Rink and T. Yurdakul (2004). "Use of a laser to detect viable but immotile spermatozoa." *Andrologia* 36(6): 366-369.

[5] Al-Malki, A., K. Alrabeeah, E. Mondou, V. Brochu-Lafontaine, S. Phillips and A. Zini (2017). "Testicular sperm aspiration (TESA)

for infertile couples with severe or complete asthenozoospermia." *Andrology* 5(2): 226-231.

[6] Al Omrani, B., N. Al Eisa, M. Javed, M. Al Ghedan, H. Al Matrafi and H. Al Sufyan (2018). "Associations of sperm DNA fragmentation with lifestyle factors and semen parameters of Saudi men and its impact on ICSI outcome." *Reprod Biol Endocrinol* 16(1): 49.

[7] Alikani, M., G. Palermo, A. Adler, M. Bertoil, M. Blake and J. Cohen (1995). "Intracytoplasmic sperm injection in dysmorphic human oocytes." *Zygote* 3(4): 283-288.

[8] Alvarez Sedó, C., M. Bilinski, D. Lorenzi, H. Uriondo, F. Noblía, V. Longobucco, E. V. Lagar and F. Nodar (2017). "Effect of sperm DNA fragmentation on embryo development: clinical and biological aspects." *JBRA Assist Reprod* 21(4): 343-350.

[9] Aman, R. R. and J. E. Parks (1994). "Effects of cooling and rewarming on the meiotic spindle and chromosomes of in vitro-matured bovine oocytes." *Biology of Reproduction* 50(1): 103-110.

[10] Anifandis, G., K. Dafopoulos, C. Messini, N. Chalvatzas and I. Messinis (2010). "Effect of the position of the polar body during ICSI on fertilization rate and embryo development." *Reproductive Sciences* 17(9): 849-853.

[11] Aydinuraz, B., E. K. Dirican, S. Olgan, O. Aksunger and O. K. Erturk (2016). "Artificial oocyte activation after intracytoplasmic morphologically selected sperm injection: A prospective randomized sibling oocyte study." *Human fertility* 19(4): 282-288.

[12] Baart, E. B., N. S. Macklon and B. J. Fauser (2009). "Ovarian stimulation and embryo quality." *Reproductive biomedicine online* 18: S45-S50.

[13] Balaban, B., B. Urman, A. Sertac, C. Alatas, S. Aksoy and R. Mercan (1998). "Oocyte morphology does not affect fertilization rate, embryo quality and implantation rate after intracytoplasmic sperm injection." *Human reproduction (Oxford, England)* 13(12): 3431-3433.

[14] Balaban, B., K. Yakin, C. Alatas, O. Oktem, A. Isiklar and B. Urman (2011). "Clinical outcome of intracytoplasmic injection of

spermatozoa morphologically selected under high magnification: a prospective randomized study." *Reproductive biomedicine online* 22(5): 472-476.

[15] Balakier, H., D. Bouman, A. Sojecki, C. Librach and J. A. Squire (2002). "Morphological and cytogenetic analysis of human giant oocytes and giant embryos." *Human reproduction* 17(9): 2394-2401.

[16] Balakier, H., A. Sojecki, G. Motamedi and C. Librach (2004). "Time-dependent capability of human oocytes for activation and pronuclear formation during metaphase II arrest." *Human reproduction* 19(4): 982-987.

[17] Baltaci, V., Ö. Ü. Ayvaz, E. Ünsal, Y. Aktaş, A. Baltacı, F. Turhan, S. Özcan and M. Sönmezer (2010). "The effectiveness of intracytoplasmic sperm injection combined with piezoelectric stimulation in infertile couples with total fertilization failure." *Fertility and sterility* 94(3): 900-904.

[18] Bartolacci, A., L. Pagliardini, S. Makieva, A. Salonia, E. Papaleo and P. Viganò (2018). "Abnormal sperm concentration and motility as well as advanced paternal age compromise early embryonic development but not pregnancy outcomes: a retrospective study of 1266 ICSI cycles." *Journal of Assisted Reproduction and Genetics* 35(10): 1897-1903.

[19] Battaglia, D. E., J. K. Koehler, N. A. Klein and M. J. Tucker (1997). "Failure of oocyte activation after intracytoplasmic sperm injection using round-headed sperm." *Fertility and sterility* 68(1): 118-122.

[20] Beck-Fruchter, R., E. Shalev and A. Weiss (2016). "Clinical benefit using sperm hyaluronic acid binding technique in ICSI cycles: a systematic review and meta-analysis." *Reproductive biomedicine online* 32(3): 286-298.

[21] Benchaib, M., V. Braun, J. Lornage, S. Hadj, B. Salle, H. Lejeune and J. F. Guérin (2003). "Sperm DNA fragmentation decreases the pregnancy rate in an assisted reproductive technique." *Human Reproduction* 18(5): 1023-1028.

[22] Benchaib, M., J. Lornage, C. Mazoyer, H. Lejeune, B. Salle and J. François Guerin (2007). "Sperm deoxyribonucleic acid

fragmentation as a prognostic indicator of assisted reproductive technology outcome." *Fertil Steril* 87(1): 93-100.

[23] Braga, D. P. d. A. F., A. S. Setti, R. C. Figueira, M. Nichi, C. D. Martinhago, A. Iaconelli Jr and E. Borges Jr (2011). "Sperm organelle morphologic abnormalities: contributing factors and effects on intracytoplasmic sperm injection cycles outcomes." *Urology* 78(4): 786-791.

[24] Buffone, M. G., E. V. Wertheimer, P. E. Visconti and D. Krapf (2014). "Central role of soluble adenylyl cyclase and cAMP in sperm physiology." *Biochimica Et Biophysica Acta (BBA)-Molecular Basis of Disease* 1842(12): 2610-2620.

[25] Caglar, G. S., F. Köster, B. Schöpper, B. Asimakopoulos, B. Nehls, N. Nikolettos, K. Diedrich and S. Al-Hasani (2007). "Semen DNA fragmentation index, evaluated with both TUNEL and Comet assay, and the ICSI outcome." *In Vivo* 21(6): 1075-1080.

[26] Carvalho, M., F. Leal, S. Mota, A. Aguiar, S. Sousa, J. Nunes and C. Calhaz-Jorge (2020). "The effect of denudation and injection timing in the reproductive outcomes of ICSI cycles: new insights into the risk of in vitro oocyte ageing." *Human reproduction* 35(10): 2226-2236.

[27] Casanovas, A., J. Ribas-Maynou, S. Lara-Cerrillo, A. R. Jimenez-Macedo, O. Hortal, J. Benet, J. Carrera and A. García-Peiró (2019). "Double-stranded sperm DNA damage is a cause of delay in embryo development and can impair implantation rates." *Fertil Steril* 111(4): 699-707.e691.

[28] Casper, R. F., J. S. Meriano, K. A. Jarvi, L. Cowan and M. L. Lucato (1996). "The hypo-osmotic swelling test for selection of viable sperm for intracytoplasmic sperm injection in men with complete asthenozoospermia." *Fertility and sterility* 65(5): 972-976.

[29] Cassuto, N. G., D. Bouret, J. M. Plouchart, S. Jellad, P. Vanderzwalmen, R. Balet, L. Larue and Y. Barak (2009). "A new real-time morphology classification for human spermatozoa: a link for fertilization and improved embryo quality." *Fertility and sterility* 92(5): 1616-1625.

[30] Cassuto, N. G., A. Hazout, D. Bouret, R. Balet, L. Larue, J. L. Benifla and G. Viot (2014). "Low birth defects by deselecting abnormal spermatozoa before ICSI." *Reproductive biomedicine online* 28(1): 47-53.

[31] Ciotti, P., L. Notarangelo, A. Morselli-Labate, V. Felletti, E. Porcu and S. Venturoli (2004). "First polar body morphology before ICSI is not related to embryo quality or pregnancy rate." *Human reproduction* 19(10): 2334-2339.

[32] De Geyter, C., C. Calhaz-Jorge, M. S. Kupka, C. Wyns, E. Mocanu, T. Motrenko, G. Scaravelli, J. Smeenk, S. Vidakovic and V. Goossens (2020). "ART in Europe, 2015: results generated from European registries by ESHRE." *Human reproduction open* 2020(1): hoz038.

[33] De Santis, L., I. Cino, E. Rabellotti, F. Calzi, P. Persico, A. Borini and G. Coticchio (2005). "Polar body morphology and spindle imaging as predictors of oocyte quality." *Reproductive biomedicine online* 11(1): 36-42.

[34] De Vincentiis, S., E. De Martino, M. G. Buffone and S. Brugo-Olmedo (2013). "Use of metaphase I oocytes matured in vitro is associated with embryo multinucleation." *Fertility and sterility* 99(2): 414-421. e414.

[35] De Vos, A., H. Van de Velde, G. Bocken, G. Eylenbosch, N. Franceus, G. Meersdom, S. Tistaert, A. Vankelecom, H. Tournaye and G. Verheyen (2013). "Does intracytoplasmic morphologically selected sperm injection improve embryo development? A randomized sibling-oocyte study." *Human reproduction* 28(3): 617-626.

[36] De Vos, A., H. Van de Velde, H. Joris and A. Van Steirteghem (1999). "In-vitro matured metaphase-I oocytes have a lower fertilization rate but similar embryo quality as mature metaphase-II oocytes after intracytoplasmic sperm injection." *Human reproduction* 14(7): 1859-1863.

[37] Dirican, E. K., A. Isik, K. Vicdan, E. Sozen and Z. Suludere (2008). "Clinical pregnancies and livebirths achieved by intracytoplasmic injection of round headed acrosomeless spermatozoa with and without oocyte activation in familial

globozoospermia: case report." *Asian journal of andrology* 10(2): 332-336.

[38] Dirican, E. K., O. D. Özgün, S. Akarsu, K. O. Akın, Ö. Ercan, M. Uğurlu, Ç. Çamsarı, O. Kanyılmaz, A. Kaya and A. Ünsal (2008). "Clinical outcome of magnetic activated cell sorting of non-apoptotic spermatozoa before density gradient centrifugation for assisted reproduction." *Journal of Assisted Reproduction and Genetics* 25(8): 375-381.

[39] Dozortsev, D., P. Nagy, S. Abdelmassih, F. Oliveira, A. Brasil, V. Abdelmassih, M. Diamond and R. Abdelmassih (2004). "The optimal time for intracytoplasmic sperm injection in the human is from 37 to 41 hours after administration of human chorionic gonadotropin." *Fertility and sterility* 82(6): 1492-1496.

[40] Dumoulin, J. C., E. Coonen, M. Bras, J. M. Bergers-Janssen, R. C. Ignoul-Vanvuchelen, L. C. van Wissen, J. P. Geraedts and J. L. Evers (2001). "Embryo development and chromosomal anomalies after ICSI: effect of the injection procedure." *Human reproduction* 16(2): 306-312.

[41] Dyer, S., G. M. Chambers, J. de Mouzon, K.-G. Nygren, F. Zegers-Hochschild, R. Mansour, O. Ishihara, M. Banker and G. D. Adamson (2016). "International Committee for Monitoring Assisted Reproductive Technologies world report: assisted reproductive technology 2008, 2009 and 2010." *Human reproduction* 31(7): 1588-1609.

[42] Ebner, T., M. Moser, M. Sommergruber, U. Gaiswinkler, O. Shebl, K. Jesacher and G. Tews (2005). "Occurrence and developmental consequences of vacuoles throughout preimplantation development." *Fertility and sterility* 83(6): 1635-1640.

[43] Ebner, T., M. Moser, M. Sommergruber, K. Jesacher and G. Tews (2004). "Complete oocyte activation failure after ICSI can be overcome by a modified injection technique." *Human reproduction* 19(8): 1837-1841.

[44] Ebner, T., M. Moser, M. Sommergruber, M. Puchner, R. Wiesinger and G. Tews (2003). "Developmental competence of oocytes showing increased cytoplasmic viscosity." *Human reproduction* 18(6): 1294-1298.

[45] Ebner, T., M. Moser, M. Sommergruber, C. Yaman, U. Pfleger and G. Tews (2002). "First polar body morphology and blastocyst formation rate in ICSI patients." *Human reproduction* 17(9): 2415-2418.

[46] Ebner, T., M. Moser and G. Tews (2006). "Is oocyte morphology prognostic of embryo developmental potential after ICSI?" *Reproductive biomedicine online* 12(4): 507-512.

[47] Ebner, T., C. Yaman, M. Moser, M. Sommergruber, O. Feichtinger and G. Tews (2000). "Prognostic value of first polar body morphology on fertilization rate and embryo quality in intracytoplasmic sperm injection." *Human reproduction* 15(2): 427-430.

[48] Ebner, T., C. Yaman, M. Moser, M. Sommergruber, K. Jesacher and G. Tews (2001). "A prospective study on oocyte survival rate after ICSI: influence of injection technique and morphological features." *Journal of Assisted Reproduction and Genetics* 18(12): 623-628.

[49] Egashira, A., M. Murakami, K. Haigo, T. Horiuchi and T. Kuramoto (2009). "A successful pregnancy and live birth after intracytoplasmic sperm injection with globozoospermic sperm and electrical oocyte activation." *Fertility and sterility* 92(6): 2037. e2035-2037. e2039.

[50] El-Nour, A. M., H. A. Al Mayman, K. A. Jaroudi and S. Coskun (2001). "Effects of the hypo-osmotic swelling test on the outcome of intracytoplasmic sperm injection for patients with only nonmotile spermatozoa available for injection: a prospective randomized trial." *Fertility and sterility* 75(3): 480-484.

[51] Esbert, M., A. Pacheco, F. Vidal, M. Florensa, M. Riqueros, A. Ballesteros, N. Garrido and G. Calderón (2011). "Impact of sperm DNA fragmentation on the outcome of IVF with own or donated oocytes." *Reprod Biomed Online* 23(6): 704-710.

[52] Esfandiari, N., H. Burjaq, L. Gotlieb and R. F. Casper (2006). "Brown oocytes: implications for assisted reproductive technology." *Fertility and sterility* 86(5): 1522-1525.

[53] Esfandiari, N., E. A. Claessens, H. Burjaq, L. Gotlieb and R. F. Casper (2008). "Ongoing twin pregnancy after rescue

intracytoplasmic sperm injection of unfertilized abnormal oocytes." *Fertility and sterility* 90(1): 199. e195-199. e197.

[54] Esfandiari, N., E. A. Ryan, L. Gotlieb and R. F. Casper (2005). "Successful pregnancy following transfer of embryos from oocytes with abnormal zona pellucida and cytoplasm morphology." *Reproductive biomedicine online* 11(5): 620-623.

[55] ESHRE (2011). "The Istanbul consensus workshop on embryo assessment: proceedings of an expert meeting." *Human reproduction* 26(6): 1270-1283.

[56] Esteves, S. C., F. Sánchez-Martín, P. Sánchez-Martín, D. T. Schneider and J. Gosálvez (2015). "Comparison of reproductive outcome in oligozoospermic men with high sperm DNA fragmentation undergoing intracytoplasmic sperm injection with ejaculated and testicular sperm." *Fertility and sterility* 104(6): 1398-1405.

[57] Falcone, P., L. Gambera, M. Pisoni, V. Lofiego, V. De Leo, L. Mencaglia and P. Piomboni (2008). "Correlation between oocyte preincubation time and pregnancy rate after intracytoplasmic sperm injection." *Gynecological Endocrinology* 24(6): 295-299.

[58] Fancsovits, P., Z. G. Tóthné, A. Murber, F. Takacs, Z. Papp and J. Urbancsek (2006). "Correlation between first polar body morphology and further embryo development." *Acta Biologica Hungarica* 57(3): 331-338.

[59] French, D. B., E. S. Sabanegh Jr, J. Goldfarb and N. Desai (2010). "Does severe teratozoospermia affect blastocyst formation, live birth rate, and other clinical outcome parameters in ICSI cycles?" *Fertility and sterility* 93(4): 1097-1103.

[60] Garor, R., Y. Shufaro, N. Kotler, D. Shefer, N. Krasilnikov, A. Ben-Haroush, H. Pinkas, B. Fisch and O. Sapir (2015). "Prolonging oocyte in vitro culture and handling time does not compensate for a shorter interval from human chorionic gonadotropin administration to oocyte pickup." *Fertility and sterility* 103(1): 72-75.

[61] Gaspard, O., P. Vanderzwalmen, B. Wirleitner, S. Ravet, F. Wenders, V. Eichel, A. Mocková, D. Spitzer, C. Jouan and V. Gridelet (2018). "Impact of high magnification sperm selection

on neonatal outcomes: a retrospective study." *Journal of Assisted Reproduction and Genetics* 35(6): 1113-1121.

[62] Ghosh, S., R. Chattopadhyay, G. Bose, A. Ganesh, S. Das and B. Chakravarty (2012). "Selection of birefringent spermatozoa under Polscope: effect on intracytoplasmic sperm injection outcome." *Andrologia* 44: 734-738.

[63] Gianaroli, L., M. C. Magli, A. P. Ferraretti, A. Crippa, M. Lappi, S. Capitani and B. Baccetti (2010). "Birefringence characteristics in sperm heads allow for the selection of reacted spermatozoa for intracytoplasmic sperm injection." *Fertility and sterility* 93(3): 807-813.

[64] Goswami, G., M. Sharma, D. Jugga and D. M. Gouri (2018). "Can intracytoplasmic morphologically selected spermatozoa injection be used as first choice of treatment for severe male factor infertility patients?" *Journal of human reproductive sciences* 11(1): 40.

[65] Greco, E., F. Scarselli, M. Iacobelli, L. Rienzi, F. Ubaldi, S. Ferrero, G. Franco, N. Anniballo, C. Mendoza and J. Tesarik (2005). "Efficient treatment of infertility due to sperm DNA damage by ICSI with testicular spermatozoa." *Human reproduction* 20(1): 226-230.

[66] Haddad, M., J. Stewart, P. Xie, S. Cheung, A. Trout, D. Keating, A. Parrella, S. Lawrence, Z. Rosenwaks and G. D. Palermo (2020). "Thoughts on the popularity of ICSI." *Journal of Assisted Reproduction and Genetics* 1-23.

[67] Halvaei, I., M. A. Khalili, M. H. Razi and S. A. Nottola (2012). "The effect of immature oocytes quantity on the rates of oocytes maturity and morphology, fertilization, and embryo development in ICSI cycles." *Journal of Assisted Reproduction and Genetics* 29(8): 803-810.

[68] Halvaei, I., M. A. Khalili, M. Soleimani and M. H. Razi (2011). "Evaluating the role of first polar body morphology on rates of fertilization and embryo development in ICSI cycles." *International journal of fertility & sterility* 5(2): 110.

[69] Hassan-Ali, H., A. Hisham-Saleh, D. El-Gezeiry, I. Baghdady, I. Ismaeil and J. Mandelbaum (1998). "Perivitelline space granularity: a sign of human menopausal gonadotrophin

overdose in intracytoplasmic sperm injection." *Human reproduction (Oxford, England)* 13(12): 3425-3430.

[70] Henkel, R., E. Kierspel, M. Hajimohammad, T. Stalf, C. Hoogendijk, C. Mehnert, R. Menkveld, W. B. Schill and T. F. Kruger (2003). "DNA fragmentation of spermatozoa and assisted reproduction technology." *Reprod Biomed Online* 7(4): 477-484.

[71] Ho, J. Y.-P., M.-J. Chen, Y.-C. Yi, H.-F. Guu and E. S.-C. Ho (2003). "The effect of preincubation period of oocytes on nuclear maturity, fertilization rate, embryo quality, and pregnancy outcome in IVF and ICSI." *Journal of Assisted Reproduction and Genetics* 20(9): 358-364.

[72] Horner, V. L. and M. F. Wolfner (2008). "Transitioning from egg to embryo: triggers and mechanisms of egg activation." *Developmental dynamics: an official publication of the American Association of Anatomists* 237(3): 527-544.

[73] Huang, C. C., D. P. Lin, H. M. Tsao, T. C. Cheng, C. H. Liu and M. S. Lee (2005). "Sperm DNA fragmentation negatively correlates with velocity and fertilization rates but might not affect pregnancy rates." *Fertil Steril* 84(1): 130-140.

[74] Huang, F.-J., S.-Y. Chang, M.-Y. Tsai, Y.-C. Lin, F.-T. Kung, J.-F. Wu and Y.-J. Lu (1999). "Relationship of the human cumulus-free oocyte maturational profile with in vitro outcome parameters after intracytoplasmic sperm injection." *Journal of Assisted Reproduction and Genetics* 16(9): 483-487.

[75] Huang, M.-T., R. K.-K. Lee, C.-H. Lu, Y.-J. Chen, S.-H. Li and Y.-M. Hwu (2015). "The efficiency of conventional microscopic selection is comparable to the hyaluronic acid binding method in selecting spermatozoa for male infertility patients." *Taiwanese Journal of Obstetrics and Gynecology* 54(1): 48-53.

[76] Imthurn, B., E. Macas, M. Rosselli and P. Keller (1996). "Endocrinology: Nuclear maturity and oocyte morphology after stimulation with highly purified follicle stimulating hormone compared to human menopausal gonadotrophin." *Human Reproduction* 11(11): 2387-2391.

[77] Jacobs, M., A. M. Stolwijk and A. M. Wetzels (2001). "The effect of insemination/injection time on the results of IVF and ICSI." *Human reproduction* 16(8): 1708-1713.
[78] Jones, K. T. (2005). "Mammalian egg activation: from Ca2+ spiking to cell cycle progression." *Reproduction* 130(6): 813-823.
[79] Kahraman, S., K. Yakın, E. Dönmez, H. Şamlı, M. Bahce, G. Cengiz, S. Sertyel, M. Şamlı and N. İmirzalıoğlu (2000). "Relationship between granular cytoplasm of oocytes and pregnancy outcome following intracytoplasmic sperm injection." *Human reproduction* 15(11): 2390-2393.
[80] Kang, Y.-N., Y.-W. Hsiao, C.-Y. Chen and C.-C. Wu (2018). "Testicular sperm is superior to ejaculated sperm for ICSI in cryptozoospermia: An update systematic review and meta-analysis." *Scientific reports* 8(1): 1-9.
[81] Khalili, M. A., M. Mojibian and A.-M. Sultan (2005). "Role of oocyte morphology on fertilization and embryo formation in assisted reproductive techniques." *Middle East Fertility Society Journal* 10(1): 72-77.
[82] Kheirollahi-Kouhestani, M., S. Razavi, M. Tavalaee, M. Deemeh, M. Mardani, J. Moshtaghian and M. Nasr-Esfahani (2009). "Selection of sperm based on combined density gradient and Zeta method may improve ICSI outcome." *Human reproduction* 24(10): 2409-2416.
[83] Kilani, S., S. Cooke and M. Chapman (2011). "Time course of meiotic spindle development in MII oocytes." *Zygote* 19(1): 55.
[84] Kim, E.-K., E.-H. Kim, E.-A. Kim, K.-A. Lee, J.-E. Shin and H. Kwon (2015). "Comparison of the effect of different media on the clinical outcomes of the density-gradient centrifugation/ swim-up and swim-up methods." *Clinical and experimental reproductive medicine* 42(1): 22.
[85] Knez, K., B. Zorn, T. Tomazevic, E. Vrtacnik-Bokal and I. Virant-Klun (2011). "The IMSI procedure improves poor embryo development in the same infertile couples with poor semen quality: a comparative prospective randomized study." *Reproductive Biology and Endocrinology* 9(1): 1-8.

[86] Kordus, R. J., R. L. Price, J. M. Davis and G. F. Whitman-Elia (2008). "Successful twin birth following blastocyst culture of embryos derived from the immotile ejaculated spermatozoa from a patient with primary ciliary dyskinesia: a case report." *Journal of Assisted Reproduction and Genetics* 25(9): 437-443.

[87] Kovačič, B., V. Vlaisavljević and M. Reljič (2006). "Clinical use of pentoxifylline for activation of immotile testicular sperm before ICSI in patients with azoospermia." *Journal of andrology* 27(1): 45-52.

[88] Kuentz, P., F. Vanden Meerschaut, E. Elinati, M. Nasr-Esfahani, T. Gurgan, N. Iqbal, F. Carré-Pigeon, F. Brugnon, S. Gitlin and J. Velez De La Calle (2013). "Assisted oocyte activation overcomes fertilization failure in globozoospermic patients regardless of the DPY19L2 status." *Human reproduction* 28(4): 1054-1061.

[89] Loutradis, D., P. Drakakis, K. Kallianidis, S. Milingos, S. Dendrinos and S. Michalas (1999). "Oocyte morphology correlates with embryo quality and pregnancy rate after intracytoplasmic sperm injection." *Fertility and sterility* 72(2): 240-244.

[90] Mangoli, V., R. Mangoli, S. Dandekar, K. Suri and S. Desai (2011). "Selection of viable spermatozoa from testicular biopsies: a comparative study between pentoxifylline and hypoosmotic swelling test." *Fertility and sterility* 95(2): 631-634.

[91] Mansour, R. T., M. A. Aboulghar, G. I. Serour, N. A. Tawab, Y. Amin and M. A. Sattar (1996). "Successful intracytoplasmic sperm injection without performing cytoplasmic aspiration." *Fertility and sterility* 66(2): 256-259.

[92] Marci, R., F. Murisier, G. L. Monte, I. Soave, A. Chanson, F. Urner and M. Germond (2013). "Clinical outcome after IMSI procedure in an unselected infertile population: a pilot study." *Reproductive health* 10(1): 1-5.

[93] Massarotti, C., S. Stigliani, A. Ramone, F. Bovis, F. Sozzi, V. Remorgida, A. Cagnacci, P. Anserini and P. Scaruffi (2021). "Occurrence of smooth endoplasmic reticulum aggregates in metaphase II oocytes: relationship with stimulation protocols and outcome of ICSI and IVF cycles." *Human reproduction.*

[94] McCulloh, D. H., J. Goorbarry, S. Shah and K. Ahmad (2011). "Oocyte lysis following intracytoplasmic sperm injection: association with measures of oocyte quality and technician performance." *Journal of Reproductive and Stem Cell Biotechnology* 2(1): 46-54.

[95] Montag, M., K. Rink, G. Delacretaz and H. Van Der Ven (2000). "Laser-induced immobilization and plasma membrane permeabilization in human spermatozoa." *Human reproduction* 15(4): 846-852.

[96] Moon, J. H., C. S. Hyun, S. W. Lee, W. Y. Son, S. H. Yoon and J. H. Lim (2003). "Visualization of the metaphase II meiotic spindle in living human oocytes using the Polscope enables the prediction of embryonic developmental competence after ICSI." *Human reproduction* 18(4): 817-820.

[97] Morton, P. C., C. S. Yoder, M. J. Tucker, G. Wright, W. D. Brockman and H. I. Kort (1997). "Reinsemination by intracytoplasmic sperm injection of 1-day-old oocytes after complete conventional fertilization failure." *Fertility and sterility* 68(3): 488-491.

[98] Nagy, Z., J. Liu, G. Joris, G. Bocken, B. Desmet, A. Van Ranst, A. Vankelecom, P. Devroey and A. Van Steirteghem (1995). "The influence of the site of sperm deposition and mode of oolemma breakage at intracytoplasmic sperm injection on fertilization and embryo development rates." *Human reproduction* 10(12): 3171-3177.

[99] Nasr-Esfahani, M., S. Razavi, A. Vahdati, F. Fathi and M. Tavalaee (2008). "Evaluation of sperm selection procedure based on hyaluronic acid binding ability on ICSI outcome." *Journal of Assisted Reproduction and Genetics* 25(5): 197-203.

[100] Navarro, P. A., M. M. de Araújo, C. M. de Araújo, M. Rocha, R. dos Reis and W. Martins (2009). "Relationship between first polar body morphology before intracytoplasmic sperm injection and fertilization rate, cleavage rate, and embryo quality." *International Journal of Gynecology & Obstetrics* 104(3): 226-229.

[101] Nordhoff, V., A. Schüring, C. Krallmann, M. Zitzmann, S. Schlatt, L. Kiesel and S. Kliesch (2013). "Optimizing TESE-ICSI

by laser-assisted selection of immotile spermatozoa and polarization microscopy for selection of oocytes." *Andrology* 1(1): 67-74.

[102] O'Neill, C., S. Cheung, A. Parrella, D. Keating, P. Xie, Z. Rosenwaks and G. D. Palermo (2020). *Relevance of oocyte morphology on ICSI outcomes.* Pick Up and Oocyte Management, Springer: 253-264.

[103] Ohlander, S., J. Hotaling, E. Kirshenbaum, C. Niederberger and M. L. Eisenberg (2014). "Impact of fresh versus cryopreserved testicular sperm upon intracytoplasmic sperm injection pregnancy outcomes in men with azoospermia due to spermatogenic dysfunction: a meta-analysis." *Fertility and sterility* 101(2): 344-349.

[104] Oleszczuk, K., A. Giwercman and M. Bungum (2016). "Sperm chromatin structure assay in prediction of in vitro fertilization outcome." *Andrology* 4(2): 290-296.

[105] Oliveira, J. B. A., M. Cavagna, C. G. Petersen, A. L. Mauri, F. C. Massaro, L. F. Silva, R. L. Baruffi and J. G. Franco (2011). "Pregnancy outcomes in women with repeated implantation failures after intracytoplasmic morphologically selected sperm injection (IMSI)." *Reproductive Biology and Endocrinology* 9(1): 1-7.

[106] Organization, W. H. (2010). "*WHO laboratory manual for the examination and processing of human semen.*"

[107] Ortega, C., G. Verheyen, D. Raick, M. Camus, P. Devroey and H. Tournaye (2011). "Absolute asthenozoospermia and ICSI: what are the options?" *Human reproduction update* 17(5): 684-692.

[108] Otsuki, J., A. Okada, K. Morimoto, Y. Nagai and H. Kubo (2004). "The relationship between pregnancy outcome and smooth endoplasmic reticulum clusters in MII human oocytes." *Human reproduction* 19(7): 1591-1597.

[109] Palermo, G., H. Joris, P. Devroey and A. C. Van Steirteghem (1992). "Pregnancies after intracytoplasmic injection of single spermatozoon into an oocyte." *The Lancet* 340(8810): 17-18.

[110] Palermo, G. D., Q. V. Neri, T. Cozzubbo and Z. Rosenwaks (2014). "Perspectives on the assessment of human sperm chromatin integrity." *Fertil Steril* 102(6): 1508-1517.

[111] Palermo, G. D., Q. V. Neri and Z. Rosenwaks (2015). "To ICSI or Not to ICSI." *Semin Reprod Med* 33(2): 92-102.

[112] Palermo, G. D., Q. V. Neri, T. Takeuchi and Z. Rosenwaks (2009). ICSI: where we have been and where we are going. *Seminars in reproductive medicine,* © Thieme Medical Publishers.

[113] Palermo, G. D., C. L. O'Neill, S. Chow, S. Cheung, A. Parrella, N. Pereira and Z. Rosenwaks (2017). "Intracytoplasmic sperm injection: state of the art in humans." *Reproduction* 154(6): F93-f110.

[114] Parmegiani, L., G. E. Cognigni, S. Bernardi, E. Troilo, W. Ciampaglia and M. Filicori (2010). ""Physiologic ICSI": hyaluronic acid (HA) favors selection of spermatozoa without DNA fragmentation and with normal nucleus, resulting in improvement of embryo quality." *Fertility and sterility* 93(2): 598-604.

[115] Parmegiani, L., G. E. Cognigni, W. Ciampaglia, P. Pocognoli, F. Marchi and M. Filicori (2010). "Efficiency of hyaluronic acid (HA) sperm selection." *Journal of Assisted Reproduction and Genetics* 27(1): 13-16.

[116] Parrella, A., M. Irani, D. Keating, S. Chow, Z. Rosenwaks and G. D. Palermo (2019). "High proportion of immature oocytes in a cohort reduces fertilization, embryo development, pregnancy and live birth rates following ICSI." *Reproductive biomedicine online* 39(4): 580-587.

[117] Parrella, A., D. Keating, S. Cheung, P. Xie, J. D. Stewart, Z. Rosenwaks and G. D. Palermo (2019). "A treatment approach for couples with disrupted sperm DNA integrity and recurrent ART failure." *Journal of Assisted Reproduction and Genetics* 36(10): 2057-2066.

[118] Patrat, C., A. Kaffel, L. Delaroche, J. Guibert, P. Jouannet, S. Epelboin, D. De Ziegler, J.-P. Wolf and P. Fauque (2012). "Optimal timing for oocyte denudation and intracytoplasmic sperm injection." *Obstetrics and gynecology international* 2012.

[119] Perrin, A., C. Coat, M. Nguyen, M. Talagas, F. Morel, J. Amice and M. De Braekeleer (2013). "Molecular cytogenetic and genetic aspects of globozoospermia: a review." *Andrologia* 45(1): 1-9.

[120] Pregl Breznik, B., B. Kovačič and V. Vlaisavljević (2013). "Are sperm DNA fragmentation, hyperactivation, and hyaluronan-binding ability predictive for fertilization and embryo development in in vitro fertilization and intracytoplasmic sperm injection?" *Fertil Steril* 99(5): 1233-1241.

[121] Ramadan, W. M., J. Kashir, C. Jones and K. Coward (2012). "Oocyte activation and phospholipase C zeta (PLCζ): diagnostic and therapeutic implications for assisted reproductive technology." *Cell Communication and Signaling* 10(1): 1-20.

[122] Rashidi, B. H., F. Sarvi, E. S. Tehrani, F. Zayeri, M. Movahedin and N. Khanafshar (2005). "The effect of HMG and recombinant human FSH on oocyte quality: a randomized single-blind clinical trial." *European Journal of Obstetrics & Gynecology and Reproductive Biology* 120(2): 190-194.

[123] Rienzi, L., F. Ubaldi, R. Anniballo, G. Cerulo and E. Greco (1998). "Preincubation of human oocytes may improve fertilization and embryo quality after intracytoplasmic sperm injection." *Human reproduction (Oxford, England)* 13(4): 1014-1019.

[124] Rienzi, L., F. M. Ubaldi, M. Iacobelli, M. G. Minasi, S. Romano, S. Ferrero, F. Sapienza, E. Baroni, K. Litwicka and E. Greco (2008). "Significance of metaphase II human oocyte morphology on ICSI outcome." *Fertility and sterility* 90(5): 1692-1700.

[125] Rienzi, L., G. Vajta and F. Ubaldi (2011). "Predictive value of oocyte morphology in human IVF: a systematic review of the literature." *Human reproduction update* 17(1): 34-45.

[126] Rita de Cássia, S. F., D. P. d. A. F. Braga, L. Semiao-Francisco, C. Madaschi, A. Iaconelli Jr and E. Borges Jr (2010). "Metaphase II human oocyte morphology: contributing factors and effects on fertilization potential and embryo developmental ability in ICSI cycles." *Fertility and sterility* 94(3): 1115-1117.

[127] Rosenbusch, B., M. Schneider, B. Gläser and C. Brucker (2002). "Cytogenetic analysis of giant oocytes and zygotes to assess their relevance for the development of digynic triploidy." *Human reproduction* 17(9): 2388-2393.

[128] Rubino, P., S. Palini, S. Chigioni, G. Carlomagno, A. Quagliariello, S. De Stefani, A. Baglioni and C. Bulletti (2015). "Improving fertilization rate in ICSI cycles by adding myoinositol to the semen preparation procedures: a prospective, bicentric, randomized trial on sibling oocytes." *Journal of assisted reproduction and genetics* 32(3): 387-394.

[129] Rubino, P., P. Viganò, A. Luddi and P. Piomboni (2016). "The ICSI procedure from past to future: a systematic review of the more controversial aspects." *Human reproduction update* 22(2): 194-227.

[130] Sá, R., M. Cunha, J. Silva, A. Luís, C. Oliveira, J. T. da Silva, A. Barros and M. Sousa (2011). "Ultrastructure of tubular smooth endoplasmic reticulum aggregates in human metaphase II oocytes and clinical implications." *Fertility and sterility* 96(1): 143-149. e147.

[131] Serhal, P., D. Ranieri, A. Kinis, S. Marchant, M. Davies and I. Khadum (1997). "Oocyte morphology predicts outcome of intracytoplasmic sperm injection." *Human reproduction (Oxford, England)* 12(6): 1267-1270.

[132] Setti, A., R. Figueira, D. Braga, T. Aoki, A. Iaconelli Jr and E. Borges Jr (2013). "Intracytoplasmic morphologically selected sperm injection is beneficial in cases of advanced maternal age: a prospective randomized study." *European Journal of Obstetrics & Gynecology and Reproductive Biology* 171(2): 286-290.

[133] Setti, A. S., D. P. d. A. F. Braga, A. Iaconelli Jr, T. Aoki and E. Borges Jr (2013). "Twelve years of MSOME and IMSI: a review." *Reproductive biomedicine online* 27(4): 338-352.

[134] Sfontouris, I. A., C. O. Nastri, M. L. Lima, E. Tahmasbpourmarzouni, N. Raine-Fenning and W. P. Martins (2015). "Artificial oocyte activation to improve reproductive outcomes in women with previous fertilization failure: a

systematic review and meta-analysis of RCTs." *Human reproduction* 30(8): 1831-1841.
[135] Shalom-Paz, E., S. Anabusi, M. Michaeli, E. Karchovsky-Shoshan, N. Rothfarb, T. Shavit and A. Ellenbogen (2015). "Can intra cytoplasmatic morphologically selected sperm injection (IMSI) technique improve outcome in patients with repeated IVF–ICSI failure? a comparative study." *Gynecological Endocrinology* 31(3): 247-251.
[136] Sheikhi, A., M. Jalali, M. Gholamian, A. Jafarzadeh, S. Jannati and N. Mousavifar (2013). "Elimination of apoptotic spermatozoa by magnetic-activated cell sorting improves the fertilization rate of couples treated with ICSI procedure." *Andrology* 1(6): 845-849.
[137] Shen, S., A. Khabani, N. Klein and D. Battaglia (2003). "Statistical analysis of factors affecting fertilization rates and clinical outcome associated with intracytoplasmic sperm injection." *Fertility and sterility* 79(2): 355-360.
[138] Shin, S. B., J. W. Cho, S.-H. Lee, K. M. Yang, C. K. Lim and H.-S. Lee (2013). "Fertilization and pregnancy potential of immature oocytes from stimulated intracytoplasmic sperm injection cycles." *Clinical and experimental reproductive medicine* 40(1): 7.
[139] Simon, L., G. Brunborg, M. Stevenson, D. Lutton, J. McManus and S. E. Lewis (2010). "Clinical significance of sperm DNA damage in assisted reproduction outcome." *Hum Reprod* 25(7): 1594-1608.
[140] Simopoulou, M., P. Giannelou, P. Bakas, L. Gkoles, T. Kalampokas, K. Pantos and M. Koutsilieris (2016). "Making ICSI safer and more effective: a review of the human oocyte and ICSI practice." *In Vivo* 30(4): 387-400.
[141] Simopoulou, M., L. Gkoles, P. Bakas, P. Giannelou, T. Kalampokas, K. Pantos and M. Koutsilieris (2016). "Improving ICSI: A review from the spermatozoon perspective." *Systems biology in reproductive medicine* 62(6): 359-371.
[142] Singh, G. (1992). "Ultrastructural features of round-headed human spermatozoa." *International journal of fertility* 37(2): 99-102.

[143] Soares, J. B., S. Glina, N. Antunes Jr, R. Wonchockier, A. G. Galuppo and F. E. Mizrahi (2003). "Sperm tail flexibility test: a simple test for selecting viable spermatozoa for intracytoplasmic sperm injection from semen samples without motile spermatozoa." *Revista do Hospital das Clínicas* 58(5): 250-253. [*Journal of Hospital das Clínicas*]

[144] Speyer, B. E., A. R. Pizzey, M. Ranieri, R. Joshi, J. D. Delhanty and P. Serhal (2010). "Fall in implantation rates following ICSI with sperm with high DNA fragmentation." *Hum Reprod* 25(7): 1609-1618.

[145] Stoddart, N. and S. Fleming (2000). "Orientation of the first polar body of the oocyte at 6 or 12 o'clock during ICSI does not affect clinical outcome." *Human reproduction* 15(7): 1580-1585.

[146] Strassburger, D., S. Friedler, A. Raziel, E. Kasterstein, M. Schachter and R. Ron-El (2004). "The outcome of ICSI of immature MI oocytes and rescued in vitro matured MII oocytes." *Human reproduction* 19(7): 1587-1590.

[147] Sun, T. C., Y. Zhang, H. T. Li, X. M. Liu, D. X. Yi, L. Tian and Y. X. Liu (2018). "Sperm DNA fragmentation index, as measured by sperm chromatin dispersion, might not predict assisted reproductive outcome." *Taiwan J Obstet Gynecol* 57(4): 493-498.

[148] Sunderam, S., D. M. Kissin, S. B. Crawford, S. G. Folger, D. J. Jamieson, L. Warner and W. D. Barfield (2015). "Assisted reproductive technology surveillance—United States, 2012." *Morbidity and Mortality Weekly Report: Surveillance Summaries* 64(6): 1-29.

[149] Sundström, P. and B. O. Nilsson (1988). "Meiotic and cytoplasmic maturation of oocytes collected in stimulated cycles is asynchronous." *Human reproduction* 3(5): 613-619.

[150] Sutter, P. D., D. Dozortsev, C. Qian and M. Dhont (1996). "Oocyte morphology does not correlate with fertilization rate and embryo quality after intracytoplasmic sperm injection." *Human reproduction* 11(3): 595-597.

[151] Ten, J., J. Mendiola, J. Vioque, J. de Juan and R. Bernabeu (2007). "Donor oocyte dysmorphisms and their influence on

fertilization and embryo quality." *Reproductive biomedicine online* 14(1): 40-48.

[152] Tesarik, J., C. Mendoza and E. Greco (2000). "The activity (calcium oscillator?) responsible for human oocyte activation after injection with round spermatids is associated with spermatid nuclei." *Fertility and sterility* 74(6): 1245-1247.

[153] Tesarik, J. and M. Sousa (1995). "Key elements of a highly efficient intracytoplasmic sperm injection technique: Ca2+ fluxes and oocyte cytoplasmic dislocation." *Fertility and sterility* 64(4): 770-776.

[154] Van Blerkom, J. (1990). "Occurrence and developmental consequences of aberrant cellular organization in meiotically mature human oocytes after exogenous ovarian hyperstimulation." *Journal of electron microscopy technique* 16(4): 324-346.

[155] Van de Velde, H., A. De Vos, H. Joris, Z. Nagy and A. Van Steirteghem (1998). "Effect of timing of oocyte denudation and micro-injection on survival, fertilization and embryo quality after intracytoplasmic sperm injection." *Human reproduction (Oxford, England)* 13(11): 3160-3164.

[156] Van der Westerlaken, L., F. Helmerhorst, J. Hermans and N. Naaktgeboren (1999). "Intracytoplasmic sperm injection: position of the polar body affects pregnancy rate." *Human reproduction* 14(10): 2565-2569.

[157] Vanden Meerschaut, F., D. Nikiforaki, S. De Gheselle, V. Dullaerts, E. Van den Abbeel, J. Gerris, B. Heindryckx and P. De Sutter (2012). "Assisted oocyte activation is not beneficial for all patients with a suspected oocyte-related activation deficiency." *Human reproduction* 27(7): 1977-1984.

[158] Verlinsky, Y., S. Lerner, N. Illkevitch, V. Kuznetsov, I. Kuznetsov, J. Cieslak and A. Kuliev (2003). "Is there any predictive value of first polar body morphology for embryo genotype or developmental potential?" *Reproductive biomedicine online* 7(3): 336-341.

[159] Vermey, B. G., M. G. Chapman, S. Cooke and S. Kilani (2015). "The relationship between sperm head retardance using

polarized light microscopy and clinical outcomes." *Reproductive biomedicine online* 30(1): 67-73.

[160] Wang, W.-H., L. Meng, R. J. Hackett, R. Odenbourg and D. L. Keefe (2001). "The spindle observation and its relationship with fertilization after intracytoplasmic sperm injection in living human oocytes." *Fertility and sterility* 75(2): 348-353.

[161] Wang, W., L. Meng, R. Hackett and D. Keefe (2001). "Developmental ability of human oocytes with or without birefringent spindles imaged by Polscope before insemination." *Human reproduction* 16(7): 1464-1468.

[162] Westlander, G., M. Barry, O. Petrucco and R. Norman (2003). "Different fertilization rates between immotile testicular spermatozoa and immotile ejaculated spermatozoa for ICSI in men with Kartagener's syndrome." *Human reproduction* 18(6): 1286-1288.

[163] Wilding, M., L. Di Matteo, S. D'Andretti, N. Montanaro, C. Capobianco and B. Dale (2007). "An oocyte score for use in assisted reproduction." *Journal of Assisted Reproduction and Genetics* 24(8): 350-358.

[164] Xia, P. (1997). "Intracytoplasmic sperm injection: correlation of oocyte grade based on polar body, perivitelline space and cytoplasmic inclusions with fertilization rate and embryo quality." *Human reproduction (Oxford, England)* 12(8): 1750-1755.

[165] Yanagida, K. (2004). "Complete fertilization failure in ICSI." *Human cell* 17(4): 187-193.

[166] Yanagida, K., H. Yazawa, H. Katayose, K. Suzuki, K. Hoshi and A. Sato (1998). "Influence of oocyte preincubation time on fertilization after intracytoplasmic sperm injection." *Human reproduction* (Oxford, England) 13(8): 2223-2226.

[167] Yavas, Y., S. Roberge, F. Khamsi, P. Shirazi, M. W. Endman and J. C. Wong (2001). "Performing ICSI using an injection pipette with the smallest possible inner diameter and a long taper increases normal fertilization rate, decreases incidence of degeneration and tripronuclear zygotes, and enhances embryo development." *Journal of Assisted Reproduction and Genetics* 18(8): 426-435.

[168] Yazawa, H., K. Yanagida, S. Hayashi and A. Sato (2009). "The oocyte activation and Ca2+ oscillation-inducing abilities of mouse and human dead (sonicated) spermatozoa." *Zygote* 17(2): 175.

[169] Yoon, S.-Y., J. H. Eum, J. E. Lee, H. C. Lee, Y. S. Kim, J. E. Han, H. J. Won, S. H. Park, S. H. Shim and W. S. Lee (2012). "Recombinant human phospholipase C zeta 1 induces intracellular calcium oscillations and oocyte activation in mouse and human oocytes." *Human reproduction* 27(6): 1768-1780.

[170] Younis, J. S., O. Radin, I. Izhaki and M. Ben-Ami (2009). "Does first polar body morphology predict oocyte performance during ICSI treatment?" *Journal of Assisted Reproduction and Genetics* 26(11): 561-567.

[171] Zanetti, B. F., D. P. d. A. F. Braga, A. S. Setti, R. d. C. S. Figueira, A. Iaconelli Jr and E. Borges Jr (2018). "Is perivitelline space morphology of the oocyte associated with pregnancy outcome in intracytoplasmic sperm injection cycles?" *European Journal of Obstetrics & Gynecology and Reproductive Biology* 231: 225-229.

In: Intracytoplasmic Sperm Injection (ICSI) ISBN: 978-1-53619-762-4
Editor: Murid Javed

Chapter 2

THE EFFECTS OF SPERM QUALITY ON EMBRYO DEVELOPMENT AFTER INTRACYTOPLASMIC SPERM INJECTION: CURRENT STATUS AND FUTURE AREAS OF INVESTIGATION

Salman Ali Aldakhilallah[1], Naif Hamdan Alharbi[1], Yousef Al Helou[2], Nafisa Ali[3] and Jaffar Ali[4,*]

[1]Department of Reproductive Endocrine and Infertility Medicine, King Fahad Medical City, Riyadh, Saudi Arabia
[2]Fakih IVF Dubai, United Arab Emirates
[3]Androcryogenics (M) Sdn Bhd, Shah Alam, Malaysia
[4]Department of IVF, Maternity and Children Hospital, Dammam, Kingdom of Saudi Arabia

ABSTRACT

Semen analysis is the first step in diagnosis of male factor infertility. Although our understanding of the spermatogenesis and

* Corresponding Author's E-mail: jaffarali.abdullah@gmail.com.

male infertility has improved over past several decades, however, more needs to done to overcome male infertility. This chapter describes how sperm are made in the testicles, various semen parameters, manual and automated semen analysis, paternal and maternal effects on semen quality of offspring and anti-sperm antibodies.

Keywords: male infertility, semen analysis, sperm count and motility, sperm DNA fragmentation, spermatogenesis, sperm quality

Introduction

Considerable strides have been made in male infertility diagnosis and treatment, however much remains to be elucidated and accomplished. Even after the advent of intracytoplasmic sperm injection (ICSI), which was a key development in male infertility treatment, the state of the art is still somewhat less than desired and unable to meet the needs of the "infertile" male. There are as yet unattained aspects in male infertility treatment that requires focus which will be reviewed in this chapter. Indeed, it is unimaginable that prior to the introduction of ICSI, a sperm count equal to or below 1 million per mL was considered sterile and useless for application in assisted reproduction technology (ART) treatment procedures. In the ensuing years after the application of ICSI was permitted it became apparent how wrong these assumptive dicta were. ICSI paved the way for considerable advances in male infertility treatment modalities such that a number of conditions of male infertility previously thought to be insurmountable were overcome enabling thousands of previously "infertile" men achieve fatherhood.

The subjectivity of routine semen analysis along with the discrepancies in the cut-off values among the different versions of World Health Organization manuals for human sperm processing has made it unreliable and confusing (Aitken, 2018). Moreover, routine manual semen analysis does not examine for normal function of spermatozoa but only provides a glimpse of it which is grossly inadequate and does no justice to study of sperm function. Semen parameters are reliant on the completeness of the ejaculated seminal sample, the normal function of accessory sex glands, the last time of sexual activity and the abstinence time and the volumes of both testes (Shen et al., 2019; Lammers et al., 2014; Ashok and Sharma 2007).

The external appearance of the sperm is an insufficient indicator of the male fecundity. The internal component of the sperm is of a great importance, which has been largely neglected in routine semen analysis for a number of years, indeed, if not decades. The external and internal components of the sperm could offer two possibilities for explaining male infertility (Tesarik et al., 2006). Sperm quality encompasses examining both external and internal components whether assessed quantitatively or qualitatively. Decreased sperm quality is thought to be detrimental for male fecundity that consequently led to increase in ART treatment (Santi et al., 2018). Moreover, in examining the quality of sperm, the health status of accessory glands and organs in the male reproductive tract that support in vivo sperm development are important. It has been believed that secretions of these glands can impact sperm quality such as sperm DNA fragmentation levels (Richthoff et al., 2002). Many factors assessing sperm quality such as routine semen parameters, sperm DNA integrity and tests used to asses it, the abstinence period, the source of sperm (ejaculatory vs. testicular), anti-sperm antibodies, maternal and paternal effects on in utero embryonic development, hormonal imbalance and even the use of microfluidic sperm sorting chips can all affect the reproductive outcome of ICSI (Abdel Raheem et al., 2013; Santi et al., 2018; Venkatesh et al., 2011; Shen et al., 2019; Esteves et al., 2015; Harvig et al., 2020; Dabbous and Atkin 2018; Cui et al., 2015; Parrella et al., 2019).

This chapter aims to examine the different factors that impact sperm quality that may have contributory effects on the potential outcomes of the ICSI treatment procedure.

Manual Semen Analysis vs Automated Semen Analysis

Semen analysis is the first method used to diagnostically assess the male fertility. The semen quality of one sample is always different from a later one. Both types help in determining whether a male has motile sperm, but it fails to predict his chance of both natural and assisted conception (Chauraisa, Sinha and Upahdyay, 2016). It also does not conclusively confirm whether the male is azoospermic (no spermatozoa in the ejaculate). Majority of the sperm in the ejaculate comes from vas deferens and distal part of the epididymis. Semen analysis does not test for sperm function. There are currently two types of semen analysis; manual semen analysis and automated/ computerized semen analysis (Lammers et al., 2014; Ashok and Sharma 2007). A comparison of both types is illustrated in Table 1.

Table 1. Comparison between manual and automated/computerized semen analysis

Manual Semen Analysis	Automated Semen Analysis
• Cheap; does not require more equipment and special slides or chips	• Expensive; requires special equipment and special slides or chips
• No programming required	• Requires experience in programming
• Subjective	• Objective
• Lack of standardization	• Standardized
• Interpersonal and inter-laboratory variations exist	• Quick and precise
• Poor repeatability	• No interpersonal and inter-laboratory variations
• No quality control beads required	• Enhanced repeatability
• Requires microscopes for analysis	• Requires quality control beads
• Feasible	• Mostly no microscopes required
• Requires expert analysis	• No expert analysis required

There is insufficient evidence that discrepancies between manual semen analysis and automated semen analysis can affect the reproductive outcome during assisted reproduction treatment procedures. However, a study has indicated that specific morphological anomalies in sperm that is correlated with high sperm DNA fragmentation can be selectively avoided using automated semen analysis during ICSI to yield better reproductive outcomes (Sivanarayana et al., 2012).

SPERM COUNT AND MOTILITY

Finding a single spermatozoan in an azoospermic male is all what it takes for a better ICSI outcome (Abdel Raheem et al., 2013). ICSI can be advantageous compared to IVF when it is related to fertilization rates for infertile men with mild oligozoospermia (<20 x 10^6/mL) in a way to prevent fertilization failure (Westerlaken et al., 2006). In cases of complete asthenozoospermia, (zero motility) using laser targeted on the tails of spermatozoa to check for its viability can be effective to obtain a pregnancy through ICSI. If the tail were curling, this would imply it is viable and should be used for ICSI (Ortega et al., 2011; Chen et al., 2017). This technique can be used for absolute asthenozoospermic patients to help couples to father a child. This technique is safe and does not harm sperm membrane or DNA integrity (Ortega et al., 2011). Likewise, the hypoosmotic sperm tail swelling test (Jeyendran and Zaneveld, 1986, Jeyendran et al., 1992) has long been used to identify viable sperm for ICSI with good outcome (Casper et al., 1996; Ali et al., 2002; Sallam et al., 2005; Stanger et al., 2010). Of interest are the findings of a meta-analysis which showed that use of mobile phones exhibits a decrease in sperm motility and vitality (Adams et al., 2014).

SPERM MORPHOLOGY

There appears to be a relationship between sperm morphology and DNA fragmentation (Jakubik-Uljasz et al., 2020) and possibly on centriolar function (Avidor-Reiss et al., 2019); two major contributors toward the developing zygote. Globozoospermia is a rare condition seen in less than 0.1% of infertile men population, which can be devastating on the couple and challenging for ART clinics. It can be characterized by both complete and partial globozoospermia with impaired acrosomal contents. Use of oocyte artificial activating agents such calcium ionophores can lead to increased fertilization, pregnancy and live birth rates in both total and partial globozoospermic males undergoing ICSI (Taylor et al., 2010; Kamiyama et al., 2012; Karaca et al., 2015). Use of hyaluronic acid binding in partial globozoospermic males undergoing ICSI may be beneficial in increasing pregnancy rate outcome (Canepa et al., 2018).

SPERM DNA DAMAGE

There are internal and external factors that damage the nuclear DNA of the sperm. The external factors damaging the DNA of the spermatozoa are numerous and include: loss of antioxidants, drugs, chemotherapy, radiation therapy, smoking, environmental toxins, high testicle temperature, varicocele, unusual ejaculation due to non-abstinence, male reproductive tract infections, male's age and the maternal epigenetic effects on future adult males (Ficarra et al., 2013; Menezo et al., 2007; Paul, Melton and Saunders 2008; Sakkas and Alvarez 2010; Sharpe 2010). The internal factors that lead to fragmentation of the DNA of spermatozoa are: inappropriate chromatin remodeling, oxidative stress and unsuccessful apoptosis (Beshay and Bukulmez 2012). The collective effect of these three internal factors might cause the DNA damage of the spermatozoa as well as individual effects to a certain degree (Aitken and De Iuliis 2010). Defects in sperm DNA integrity might be present despite normal semen parameters; however, sperm DNA damage adversely affects pregnancy and increases risk of miscarriage (Tan et al., 2019). Infertile males with high sperm DNA fragmentation index (DFI) undergoing ICSI tend to have a significantly elevated pregnancy and implantation rates than those that has conventional IVF (Chi et al., 2017). Two meta-analyses using receiver operator characteristics curves considering all datasets and four assays (SCSA, TUNEL, SCD and Comet) have pinpointed a threshold for sperm DNA fragmentation of 20% to distinguish between fertile and infertile males with 97% sensitivity and 86% specificity (Santi et al., 2018).

There are currently four possible mechanisms by which the DNA gets damaged during the synthesis or storage of spermatozoa. The first mechanism occurs by apoptosis during spermatogenesis. The second mechanism occurs when there is replacement of sperm's chromatin with protamine during spermiogenesis. The third mechanism occurs due to damage by oxygen reactive species when the sperm is transported via the seminiferous tubules in the epididymis (Figure 1). The fourth mechanism occurs by internal caspases and endonucleases in the sperm (Sakkas and Alvarez 2010). Of these four possible mechanisms, oxidative stress is the most probable cause of DNA fragmentation of spermatozoa (Koppers et al., 2011), and endonucleases the least likely (Perry et al., 1999).

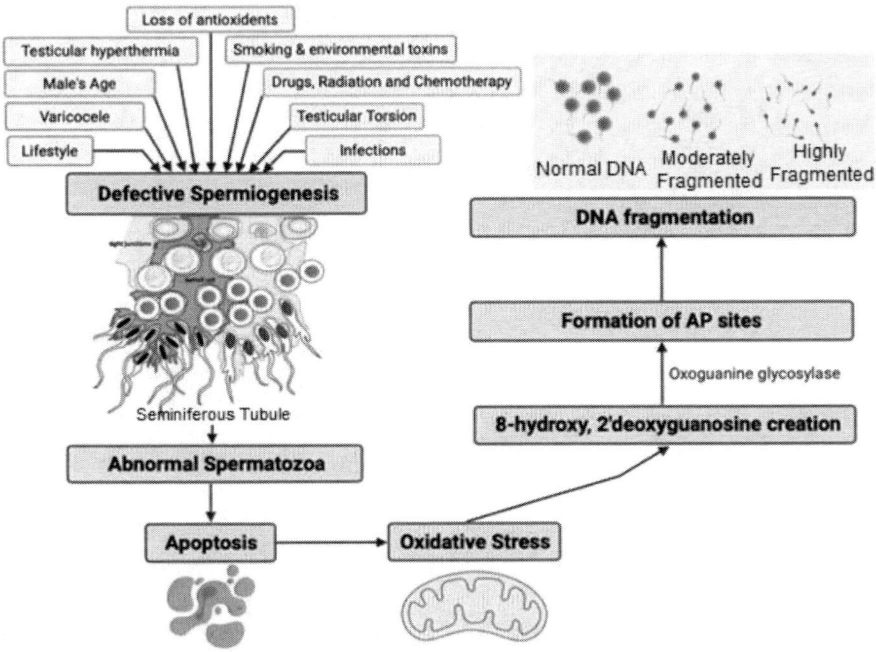

Figure 1. An overall representation of the steps involved in spermatozoa DNA fragmentation when external factors interfere with late spermiogenesis.

Defective apoptosis may result in high numbers of nonviable spermatozoa. Apoptosis is defined as genetically programmed cell death. In normal circumstances early in human development, this programmed cell death plays an important role in constructing the proper Sertoli cell ratio to the germ cell. During adult lifetime, apoptosis is still involved in assuring that the previously selected germ cells are highly trustworthy of producing the most viable spermatozoa (Aitken and Baker, 2013). Normally, factors, that favor survival of the spermatozoa, will stimulate an antiapoptotic enzyme called phosphatidlinositide 3-kinase (PI3 kinase). PI3 kinase then will lead to the phosphorylation of the serine/threonine residues in a molecule called phosphatidylinositol (3, 4, 5)-triphosphate (PIP3) (Koppers et al., 2011). After that, PIP3 will be bound to another kinase of a same kind called AKT. The phosphorylation of AKT will promote the viability of the spermatozoa as well as the intrinsic inactivation of apoptotic factors like Bcl-2 associated death promoter (BAD). There are three isoforms of AKT, but only two are found in the testes; AKT1 and AKT2. AKT1 is the predominant isoform found in the sperm, especially in the mid-piece where the fate of the cell in the mitochondria is established (Figure 2, Koppers et al., 2011). A dephosphorylation of AKT will eliminate the mechanism protect against apoptosis.

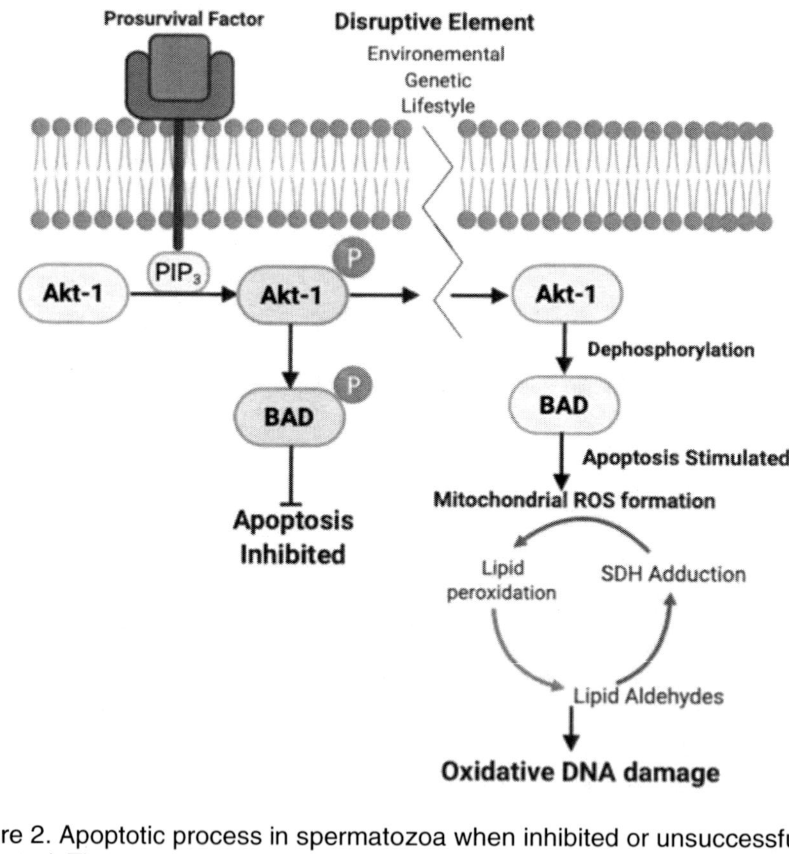

Figure 2. Apoptotic process in spermatozoa when inhibited or unsuccessfully activated. The spermatozoa is viable when AKT-1 is phosphorylated and vice versa.

Hence, this abortive apoptosis will not be for the benefit of the sperm. The high levels of polyunsaturated fatty acids (PUFA) are involved in the stimulation of oxidative stress which enhances lipid peroxidation. The latter will then form lipid aldehydes (Figure 2, Koppers et al., 2011). Use of density gradient centrifugation filters out apoptotic spermatozoa, thus, preventing any negative effects on fertilization and pregnancy rate for males undergoing ICSI (Zorn et al., 2012).

When the spermatozoa are deposited inside the female reproductive tract, they are under the influence of a maturation process called capacitation. This process appears to be active even inside the epididymis of the male reproductive tract (Bailey et al., 2010).

This process acts to supply the travelling spermatozoa with the required enzymes and nutrients to survive their journey. The chemical process by which capacitation occurs is still not known. However, it has been shown that there is cholesterol efflux from the sperm membrane by peroxynitrite (ONOO-) to form oxysterols (Bailey et al., 2010). There is also an augmented tyrosine phosphorylation (Figure 3). This process appears to follow a redox reaction and tends to favour a small number of reactive oxygen species. Hence, reduced antioxidant activity or increased production of reactive oxygen species will likely lead to DNA damage (Bailey et al., 2010).

Abnormal packaging of chromatin is also likely to cause problems, especially with more mature spermatozoa. Chromatin remodelling occurs during the process of spermiogenesis. Topoisomerase IIB aids in the replacement of histone with protamine (Ward, 2011), introducing double strand breaks in the DNA. Infertile males tend to have looser chromatin than their fertile counterparts. Protamine-bound chromatin tends to be more supercoiled than histone-bound chromatin. Disulphide bonds in sperm, which occur between cysteine residues, help to better compact sperm chromatin (Simon et al., 2011). However, when human spermatogonia become more mature, double strand breaks are formed transiently (Marcon and Boissonneault. 2004). Human sperm contain two types of protamine; Protamine 1 and Protamine 2. Unlike other species, human sperm retains up to 15% of histones. (Fuentes-Mascorro and Rosado, 2009). Sperm motility, concentration and vitality are affected when the expression of Protamine 2 is reduced by inhibin B (Aklam et al., 2016).

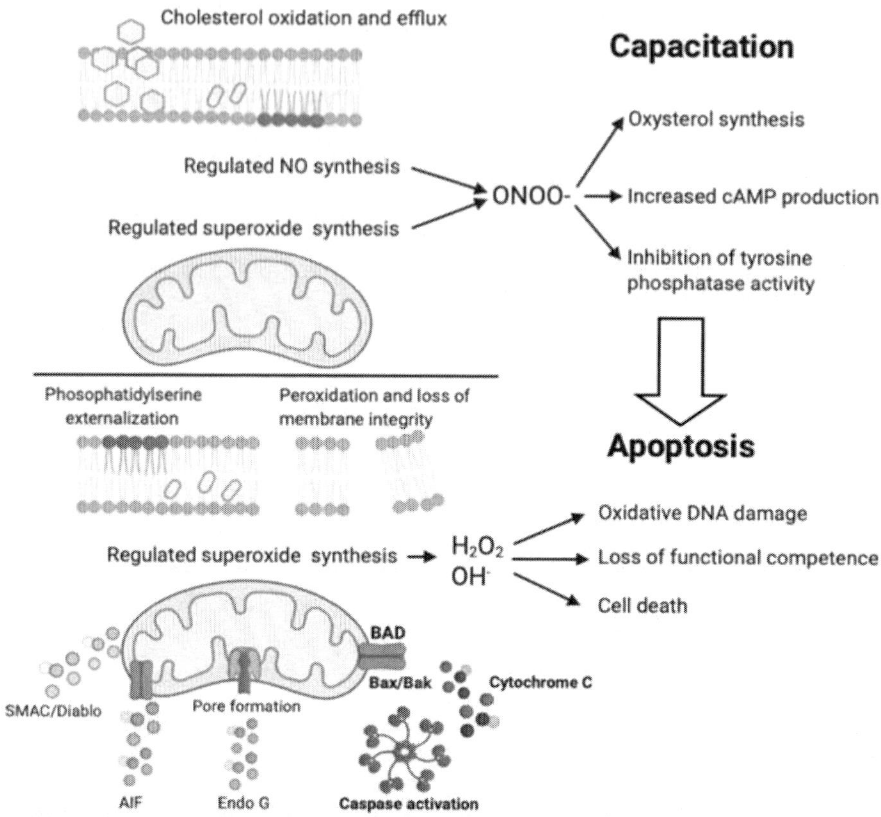

Figure 3. Sperm capacitation and its relationship with apoptosis of spermatozoa.

Oxidative stress is defined as an imbalance between antioxidant levels and reactive oxygen species; mainly affecting the epididymal transit and post ejaculation. Oxidative stress is induced by apoptosis. Hydrogen peroxide is the by-product of oxidative stress. Hydrogen peroxide is involved in the formation of 8-hydroxy-2'-deoxyguanosine (8OHdG) in the DNA backbone (Aitken et al., 2013; Mahfouz et al., 2010; Sakkas and Alvarez 2010). The repairing capacity of sperm by the enzyme oxoguanineglycosylase (OGGI) will remove 8OHdG, but in turn OGGI will introduce an abasic site (AP site) and a single strand break. An abasic site indicates a position in the DNA backbone that lacks both pyrimidine and purine bases. Subsequently, the introduction of an abasic site will make the DNA more susceptible to acid hydrolysis. The high levels of polyunsaturated fatty acids (PUFA) are involved upon the stimulation of oxidative stress in enhancing lipid peroxidation. The latter will then form lipid aldehydes (Koppers et al., 2011). Increased reactive oxygen species in semen is linked to reduced motility, abnormal acrosome reaction and male infertility (Cocuzza et al., 2007).

It has been shown that endonucleases are not involved in DNA damage for two reasons. Firstly, some endonucleases such as DNase I are too bulky to reach the genome through the chromatin. The second reason is the fact that endonucleases are trapped inside the mid-piece, separated in compartments (Aitken et al., 2013). A study has shown that endonucleases embedded inside the chromatin of sperm might possibly be involved in DNA fragmentation (Perry et al., 1999).

Oocyte-Sperm Interactions on Sperm Quality

The sperm to ova relationship is also important, because the ovum has the capacity to repair damages in the DNA of the sperm. A study has shown that ova from younger females tended to repair sperm DNA damage more effectively than ova from older females (Meseguer et al., 2011). Another study has also shown that a full oocyte-cumulus complex has a better capacity to repair sperm DNA damage than ova with no cumulus cells (Abu-Hassan et al., 2006).

Abstinence Period

Reducing the abstinence interval from 3-7 days to 1-3 hours has led to improvements in semen parameters and quality (Shen et al., 2019). While semen volumes tended to be lower, the reduced abstinence period led to increased implantation, clinical pregnancy, and live birth rates in both fresh and frozen cycles. Additionally, the reduced abstinence period demonstrated a significant decrease in sperm DNA fragmentation (Shen et al., 2019). Another study has demonstrated that a reduced abstinence period in normozoospermic males after 24 hours (with four repeated ejaculates) led to a significantly lower rate of sperm DNA fragmentation by 25% (Gosalvez et al., 2011). Moreover, a reduced abstinence period in different normozoospermic young males who submitted an ejaculate after 3 hours, coupled with density gradient for sperm selection, showed a further significant decrease in the rate of sperm DNA fragmentation by 44% (Gosalvez et al., 2011). This implies that ejaculate in patients undergoing ICSI should have a reduced abstinence period for better outcomes in younger patients. Another study looked at subsequent ejaculates 3 hours from the first sample. There was a significant increase in sperm concentration, motility, and morphology (Ragheb et al., 2018).

Sperm Source (Ejaculatory vs. Testicular)

Meta-analysis of testicular sperm retrieved from cryptozoospermia undergoing ICSI exhibited increase in the number of high quality embryos, implantation, and clinical pregnancy rates (Kang et al., 2018). Another study has shown that testicular sperm retrieved from oligozoospermic males (aged between 33-42) undergoing ICSI tended to have a significant decrease in sperm DNA fragmentation, miscarriage rates and a significant increase in live births compared with ejaculated sperm from oligozoospermic males (Esteves et al., 2015). Furthermore, this study showed that testicular sperm from males undergoing ICSI with high sperm DNA fragmentation led to improved reproductive outcomes compared with ejaculated sperm from their counterparts (Esteves et al., 2015).

Paternal and Maternal Effects on Sperm Quality of Offspring

Paternal smoking habits at the time of pregnancy can lead to a 50% decrease in sperm concentration and total sperm count (Axelsson et al., 2018; Harvig et al., 2020). Increased paternal age (> 40 yr) is related to increased assisted conception failure, chromosomal aneuploidies, risk of birth defects and childhood cancers (Bregh et al., 2019). The Yq microdeletions, specifically in the azoospermia factor c locus, are believed to be a major cause for impairing spermatogenesis, which might be transmitted to offspring through ICSI. Males with severe oligozoospermia and azoospermia diagnosed with Y chromosomal microdeletions (AZFc and AZFb loci) can bear children through ICSI with good outcomes (Liu et al., 2017; Xi et al., 2019).

Maternal high coffee consumption during pregnancy has been found to significantly harm the reproductive function of the male offspring, and reduce their semen quality (Cirillo et al., 2011). Maternal high stress levels during first trimester of pregnancy are linked to decreased sperm count and semen volume of adult sons (Brauner et al., 2019). Maternal smoking during pregnancy can lead to decreased sperm quality of the male offspring (Jensen et al., 2004; Ravnborg et al., 2011; Axelsson et al., 2018). Maternal high alcohol consumption during pregnancy tends to have a deleterious effect on semen quality and Sertoli cell function of male offspring (Ramlau-Hansen et al., 2010).

Hormonal Imbalance

Homeostatic state of circulating bodily hormones is crucial for reproductive functions. Hyperprolactinemia; caused by prolactinomas, have a deteriorating effect on male fecundity. Elevated serum prolactin levels inhibit the secretions of the anterior pituitary gonadotropic cells (Dabbous and Atkin, 2018). Indirectly, this will have an adverse effect on spermatogenesis by reducing follicular stimulating hormone (FSH). This abnormal condition is present in approximately 1% of the global population. Hence, this condition is often overlooked in patients and can result in severe oligoasthenozoospermia. The majority of these patients does not require ICSI and should first be treated with dopamine agonists such as Cabergoline, Bromocriptine or Quinagolide on a regimen varying from 2 to 24 months (Dabbous and Atkin, 2018).

Hypothyroidism is another hormonal imbalance that affects male fertility characterized by decreased levels of serum T3 and T4 and elevated levels of thyroid stimulating hormone (TSH). This correlates with decreased circulating sex binding globulin and free testosterone levels, which can lead to reduced morphology in a majority of cases. Sperm motility, and in short periods, semen volume are also affected (Vignera and Vita 2018; Alahmar, Dutta and Sengupta, 2019). The T3 hormone is important for testosterone synthesis and normal testicular function. Hypothyroidism might correlate with both decreased testicular oxidative defense and increased oxidative stress. However, there is insufficient data to support these claims in humans, and have only been studied in rat. Hypothyroidism should be treated with Levothyroxine (synthetic T4) (Vignera and Vita, 2018; Alahmar, Dutta and Sengupta, 2019).

Anti-Sperm Antibody

Anti-sperm antibody (ASA) is an immunological response found in 5-15% of the infertile male population and less than 2% in the fertile male population. Both seminal and serum ASA can impair spermatogenesis, sperm transport, implantation, preimplantation embryo growth, gamete cellular communications and lastly the developing fetus. A systemic meta-analysis has indicated that semen ASA positive cohort is significantly related to delayed liquefaction, reduced sperm concentration and decreased progressive motility (a + b) (Cui et al., 2015). Another study has shown that the ASA positive cohort with ICSI exhibited similar success rates to their negative cohort. ASA-positive males undergoing ICSI had higher pregnancy and live birth rates compared to ASA-positive males undergoing IVF (Lu et al., 2019).

Microfluidics

Microfluidics devices have recently received more attention in the field of Assisted Reproduction. Microfluidics devices are being used non-invasively for sorting normal spermatozoa in terms of motility and morphology without the need for centrifugation (Quin et al., 2018). Spermatozoa in vivo normally swim through the cervical mucus which acts as a filter, which can be replicated using microfluidic systems. Microfluidic sperm sorting chips enhance sperm quality and ICSI outcome (Parrella et al., 2019). A study showed that microfluidic sperm sorting chips lead to improved motility, morphology and reduced sperm DNA fragmentation (Quin et al., 2018). It was also found to be efficient for couples experiencing recurrent implantation failure. However, the drawback of this study was having a small sample size (Parrella et al., 2019). Moreover, a randomized controlled trial is required to validate the findings for a more robust and meaningful utilization of microfluidic devices.

CONCLUSION

The sperm with high quality internal and external components are crucial for better ICSI outcomes. However, the current tests for determination of sperm quality are invasive and destructive. Consequently, the sperm in the specimen tested are damaged rendering them useless for use in the ICSI procedure with the exception of specimen investigated using the microfluidic technique and PICSI dishes. In other words, although current methods of investigation offer the means to determine the causes of infertility in an individual but it does not provide the means to identify normal healthy unaffected sperm in the sample tested that could be utilized for ICSI because of the destructive nature of available techniques of diagnosis and investigation. Obviously, there is a need to develop more robust, non-destructive, quality controlled, standardized, safe, and reliable techniques of high specificity and sensitivity for the identification and selection of normal sperm from a sample of semen of mixed population of normal and abnormal sperm. When such useful techniques have been developed, they will enable the selection of sperm of the highest quality to assist infertile couples fulfil their aspirations for parenthood. Moreover, such assays need to be economically affordable and readily available to all infertile couples.

References

[1] Abdel-Raheem, A., Rushwan, N., Garaffa, G., Zacharakis, E., Doshi, A., Heath, C., Serhal, P., Harper, J. C., Christopher, N. A. and Ralph, D., (2013), Factors influencing intracytoplasmic sperm injection (ICSI) outcome in men with azoospermia, *BJU Internat,* 112 (2), 258-264.

[2] Abu-Hassan, D., Koester, F, Shoepper, B., Schultze-Mosgau, A., Asimakopoulos, B., Diedrich, K., Al-Hasani, S., (2006), 'Comet assay of cumulus cells and spermatozoa dna status, and the relationship to oocyte fertilization and embryo quality following ICSI'. *Reprod BioMed Online,* 12(4), 447-452.

[3] Adams, J. A., Galloway, T. S., Mondal, D, Esteves, S. C., Mathews, F., (2014), 'Effect of mobile telephones on sperm quality: a systemic review and meta-analysis'. *Environ Internat,* 70, 106-112.

[4] Agarwal, A., Allamaneni, S. S. R., (2005), 'Sperm DNA damage assessment: a test whose time has come', *Fertil Steril,* 84(4), 850-853.

[5] Agarwal, A., Sharma, R. K., (2006), Automation is the key to standardized semen analysis using the automated sqa-v sperm quality analyzer. *Fertil Steril,* 87(1), 156-162.

[6] Agbaje, I. M., McVicar, C. M., Schock, B. C., McClure, N., Atkinson, A. B., Rogers, D., Lewis, S. E. M., (2008), Increased concentrations of the oxidative DNA adduct 7,8-dihydro-8-oxo-2-deoxyguanosine in the germ line of men with type 1 diabetes, *Reprod BioMed Online,* 16 (3), 401-409.

[7] Aitken, R. J., (2018), Not every sperm is sacred; a perspective on male infertility, *Mol Human Reprod,* 24(6), 287-298.

[8] Aitken, R. J., Bronson, R., Smith, T. B. De Iuliis, G. N. (2013), The source and significance of DNA damage in human spermatozoa; a commentary on diagnosis strategies and straw man fallacies, *Mol Human Reprod,* 19(8):475-485.

[9] Aitken, R. J., Baker, M. A., (2013), Causes and consequences of apoptosis in spermatozoa; contributions to infertility and impacts on development, *Internat J Dev Biol,* 58, 265-272.

[10] Aitken, R. J., De Iuliis, G. N., (2010), On the possible origins of dna damage in human spermatozoa, *Mol Human Reprod,* 16 (1), 3-13.

[11] Akmal, M., Aulanni'am, A., Widodo, M. A., Sumitro, S. B., Purnomo, B. B., Widodo 2016, 'The important role of protamine in spermatogenesis and quality of sperm: a mini review', *Asia Pacific J Reprod,* 5(5), 357-360.

[12] Alahmar, A., Dutta, S., Sengupta, P., (2019), Thyroid hormones in male reproduction and infertility, *Asian Pacific J Reprod,* 8(5), 203-210.

[13] Ali, J., Rahbar, S., Burjaq, H. and Shahata M. A. M. 2002. Case Report: Pregnancies and births from embryos generated from oocytes fertilized by stump tail spermatozoa. *MEFS. J.* 7(3):1-4

[14] Avidor-Reiss T., Mazur M., Fishman E. L., Sindhwani P. 2019. The Role of Sperm Centrioles in Human Reproduction – The Known and the Unknown. *Front Cell Dev Biol.* 2019; 7:188 (p.1-15).

[15] Axelsson, J., Sabra, S., Rylander, L., Rignell-hydbom, A., Lindh, C. H. Giwercman, A. (2018), Association between paternal smoking at the time of pregnancy and the semen quality in sons, *Plos One,* 21;13(11):e0207221.

[16] Babazadeh, Z., Razavi, S., Tavalaee, M., Deemeh, M. R., Shahidi, M. Nasr-Esfahani, M. H. (2010), Sperm DNA damage and its relation with leukocytes DNA damage', *Reprod Toxicol,* 29, 120-124.

[17] Bailey, J. L., (2010), Factors regulating sperm capacitation', *Sys Biol Reprod Med,* 58, 770-777.

[18] Belloc, S., Benkhalifa, M., Junca, A. M., Dumont, M., Bacrie, P. C., Menezo, Y. (2009). Paternal age and sperm DNA decay: discrepancy between chromomycin and aniline blue staining, *Reprod BioMed Online,* 19(2), 264-269.

[19] Bergh, C., Pinborg, A., Wennerholm, U., (2019), Paternal age and child outcomes, *Fertil Steril,* 111 (6), 1036-1046.

[20] Beshay, V. E., Bukulmez, O., (2012), Sperm DNA damage: how relevant is it clinically?', *Current Opinion Urol*, 24(3), 172-179.

[21] Brauner, E. V., Hansen, A. M., Doherty, D. A., Dickinson, J. E., Handelsman, D. J., Hickey, M., Skakkebak, N. E., Juul, A., Hart,

R., (2019), The association between in-utero exposure to stressful life events during pregnancy and male reproductive function in a cohort of 20-year-old offspring: the raine study, *Human Reprod,* 34(7), 1345-1355.

[22] Bungum, M., Bungum, L., Lynch, K. F., Wedlund, L., Humaidan, P., Giwercman, A. (2012), Spermatozoa DNA damage measured by sperm chromatin structure assay (SCSA) and birth characteristics in children conceived by IVF and ICSI', *Internat J Androl,* 35, 485-490.

[23] Canepa, P., Casciano, I., Leo, C. D., Massarotti, C., Anserini, P., Remorgida, V. Scaruffi, P. (2018), A successful healthy childbirth and an ongoing evolutive pregnancy in a case of partial globozoospermia by hyaluronic acid sperm selection', *Andrologia,* 51(2):e13178.

[24] Casper, R. F., Meriano, J. S., Jarvi, K. A., Cowan, L., Lucato, M. L. 1996. The hypo-osmotic swelling test for selection of viable sperm for intracytoplasmic sperm injection in men with complete asthenozoospermia. *Fertil Steril.* 1996; 65(5):972-976

[25] Chaurasia, A. K., Sinha, A. K., Upahdyay, P. (2016), Comparison of semen analysis by manual and automated method, *J Pathol Nepal,* 6, 990-993.

[26] Chen, H., Feng, G., Zhang, B., Zhou, H., Shu, J., Gan, X. (2017), A successful pregnancy using completely immotile but viable frozen-thawed spermatozoa selected by laser, *Clin Exptl Reprod Med,* 44(1), 52-55.

[27] Chi, H., Kim, S., Kim, Y., Park, J., Yoo, C., Park, I., Sun, H., Kim, J., Lee, K., Park, H. (2017), ICSI significantly improved the pregnancy rate of patients with a high sperm DNA fragmentation index, *Clin Exptl Reprod Med,* 44(3), 132-140.

[28] Cirillo, P. M., Cohen, B. A., Kirgbaum, N. Y., Lee, M., Brazil, C. Facor-litvak, P., (2011), Effect of maternal coffee, smoking and drinking behaviour on adult son's semen quality: prospective evidence from the child health and development studies, *J Dev Origins Health Dis,* 2(6), 375-386.

[29] Cocuzza, M., Sikka, S. C., Athayde, K. S. Agarwal, A. (2007), Clinical relevance of oxidative stress and sperm chromatin

damage in male infertility: an evidence-based analysis, *Internat Brazilian J Urol,* 33(5), 603-621.

[30] Cui, D., Han, G., Shang, Y., Liu, C., Xia, L., Li, L., Yi, S., (2015), Antisperm antibodies in infertile men and their effect on semen parameters: a systemic review and meta-analysis, *Clin Chim Acta,* 444, 29-36.

[31] Dabbous, Z., Atkin S. L., (2018), Hyperprolactinaemia in male infertility: clinical case scenarios, *Arab J Urol,* 16, 44-52.

[32] Enciso, M., Piecezenik, G., Cohen, J. Wells, D. (2012), Development of a novel synthetic oligopeptide for the detection of DNA damage in human spermatozoa', *Human Reprod,* 27(8), 2254-2266.

[33] Esteves, S. C., Martin, F. S., Martin, P. S., Schneider, D. T. Gosalves, J. (2015), Comparison of reproductive outcome in oligozooseprmic men with high sperm DNA fragmentation undergoing intracytoplasmic sperm injection with ejaculated and testicular sperm', *Fertil Steril,* 104(6), 1398-1405.

[34] Fernandez, J. L., Muriel, L., Rivero, M. T., Goyanes, V., Vazquez, R. Alvarez, J. G., (2003), The sperm chromatin dispersion test: a simple method for the determination of sperm DNA fragmentation, *J Androl,* 24(1), 59-66.

[35] Ficarra, V., Crestani, A., Novara, G., Mirone, V., (2013), Varicocele repair for infertility: what is the evidence?, *Curr Opin Urol,* 22(6), 489-494.

[36] Fuentes-mascorro, G., Serrano, H., Rosado, A., (2000), Sperm chromatin, *Arch Androl,* 45(3), 215-225.

[37] Garrido, N., Remohi, J., Martinez-Conejero, J. A., Gracia-Herrero, S., Pellicer, A. Meseguer, M., (2008), Contribution of sperm molecular features to embryo quality and assisted reproduction success, *Reprod BioMed Online,* 17(6), 855-865.

[38] Gosalvez, J., Martinez, M. G., Fernandez, C. L., Fernandez, J. L. Sanchez-Martin, P., (2011), Shorter abstinence decreases sperm deoxyribonucleic acid fragmentation in ejaculate, *Fertil Steril,* 96(5), 1083-1086.

[39] Harvig, K. K., Hoyer, B. B., Giwercman, A., Hougaard, K. S., Ramlau-Hansen, C. H., Specht, I. O., Toft, G., Bonde, J. P., Tottenborg, S. S., (2020), Fetal exposure to paternal smoking and

semen quality in the adult son', *Androl,* pp. 1-9. doi: 10.1111/andr.12782.

[40] Henkel, R., Kierspel, E., Hajimohammad, M., Stalf, T., Hoogendijk, C., Mehnert, C., Menkveld, R., Schill, W., Kruger, T. F., (2003), DNA fragmentation of spermatozoa and assisted reproduction technology, *Reprod BioMed Online,* 7(4), 477-484.

[41] Hughes, M. C., Lewis, S. E. M., McKelvey-Martin, V. J., Thompson, W., (1996), A comparison of baseline and induced DNA damage in human spermatozoa from fertile and infertile men, using a modified comet assay, *Mol Human Reprod,* 2(8), 613-619.

[42] Jakubik-Uljasz J, Gill K, Rosiak-Gill A, Malgorzata Piasecka M. 2020. Relationship between sperm morphology and sperm DNA dispersion. *Transl Androl Urol.* 2020; 9(2): 405–415.

[43] Jensen, T. K., Jorgensen, N., Punab, M., Haugen, T. B., Suominen, J., Zilaitiene, B., Horte, A., Andersen, A. G., Carlsen, E., Magnus, O., Matulevicius, V., Nermoen, I., Vierula, M., Keiding, N., Toppari, J., Skakkebaek, N. E., (2004), Association of in utero exposure to maternal smoking with reduced semen quality and testis size in adulthood: a cross-sectional study of 1,770 young men from the general population in five European countries, *Am J Epidemiol,* 150(1), 49-58.

[44] Jeyendran R. S., Zaneveld L. J. D. 1986, Human sperm hypoosmotic swelling test. Fertil Steril 46: 151-152.

[45] Kamiyama, H., Shimizu, T., Oki, T., Asada, T., Araki, Y., Araki, Y., (2012), Successful delivery following intracytoplasmic sperm injection with calcium ionphore a23187 oocyte activation in a partially globozoospermic patient, *Reprod Med Biol,* 11, 159-164.

[46] Kang, Y., Hsiao, Y., Chen, C., Wu, C. C., (2018), Testicular sperm is superior to ejaculated sperm for ICSI in cryptozoospermia: an update systemic review and meta-analysis, *Scientific Rep,* 8(1), 7874.

[47] Karaca, N., Akpak, Y. K., Oral, S., Durmus, T. Yilmaz, R., (2015), A successful healthy childbirth in a case of total globozospermia with oocyte activation by calcium ionphore, *J Reprod Infertil,* 16(2), 116-120.

[48] Kim, H., Kang, M. J., Kim, S. A., Oh, S. K., Kim, J., Ku, S. Y., Kim, S. H., Moon, S. Y., Choi, Y. M., (2013), The utility of sperm dna damage assay using toluidine blue and aniline blue staining in routine semen analysis, *Korean Soc Reprod Med,* 40 (1), 23-28.

[49] Koppers, A. J., Mitchell, L. A., Wang, P., Lin, M. Aitken, R. J. (2011), Phosphoinositide 3-kinase signalling pathway involvement in a truncated apoptotic cascade associated with motility loss and oxidative DNA damage in human spermatozoa', *Biochem J,* 436, 687-698.

[50] Lammers, J., Splingart, C., Barriere, P., Jean, M., Freour, T., (2014), Double-blind prospective study comparing two automated sperm analyzers versus manual semen assessment, *J Assist Reprod Genet,* 31, 35-43.

[51] Liu, X., Wang, R., Fu, Y., Luo, L., Guo, W., Liu, R. Z., (2017), Outcomes of intracytoplasmic sperm injection in oligozoospermic men with y chromosome azf b or azf c microdeletions', *Andrologia,* vol. 49(1), e12602.

[52] Lu, Z., Li, X., Wang, S., Yang, X., Xu, Y., Huang, L., Liu, J., Cai, F., Chen, Z., (2019), Success rates in vitro fertilization versus intracytoplasmic sperm injection in men with serum anti-sperm antibodies: a consecutive cohort study, *Asian J Androl,* 21, 473-477.

[53] Mahfouz, R. Z., Du Plessis, S. S., Aziz, N., Sharma, R., Sabanegh, E. Agrawal, A., (2010), Sperm viability, apoptosis, and intracellular reactive oxygen species levels in human spermatozoa before and after induction of oxidative stress', *Fertil Steril,* 93(3), 814-820.

[54] Marchesi, D. E., Biederman, H., Ferrara, S., Hershlag, A., Feng, H. L., (2010), The effect of semen processing on sperm dna integrity: comparison of two techniques using novel toluidine blue assay', *Eur J Obstet Gynecol Reprod Biol,* 151, 176-180.

[55] Marcon, L., Boissonneault, G., (2004), Transient DNA strand breaks during mouse and human spermiogenesis new insights in stage specificity and link to chromatin remodelling, *Biol Reprod,* 70, 910-918.

[56] Menezo, Y. J. R., Hazout, A., Panteix, G., Robert, F., Rollet, J., Cohen-Bacrie, P., Chapuis, F., Clement, P., Benkhalifa, M.,

(2007), Antioxidants to reduce sperm DNA fragmentation: an unexpected adverse effect, *Reprod BioMed Online,* 14(4), 418-421.

[57] Meseguer, M., Santiso, R., Garrido, N., Gracia-Herrero, S., Remohi, J., Frenandez, J. L. (2011), Effect of sperm dna fragmentation on pregnancy outcome depends on oocyte quality, *Am Soc Reprod Med,* 95(1), 124-128.

[58] Mitchell, L. A., De Iuliis, G. N. Aitken, R. J. (2010), The tunel assay consistently underestimates DNA damage in human spermatozoa and is influenced by DNA compaction and cell vitality: development of an improved methodology, *Internat J Androl,* 34, 2-13.

[59] Ni, Z., Liu, Y., Shen, H., Chia, S. E. Ong, C. N., (1997), Does the increase of 8-hydroxydeoxyguanosine lead to poor sperm quality?, *Mutation Res,* 381, 77-82.

[60] Oger, I., Cruz, C. D., Panteix, G. Menezo, Y. (2003), Evaluating human sperm DNA integrity: relationship between 8-hydroxydeoxyguanosine quantification and the sperm chromatin structure assay, *Zygote,* 11, 367-371.

[61] Ortega, C., Verheyen, G., Raick, D., Camus, M., Devroey, P., Tournaye, H. (2011), Absolute asthenozoospermia and ICSI: what are the options', *Human Reprod Update,* 17(5), 684-692.

[62] Ovari, L., Sati, L., Stronk, J., Borsos, A., Ward, D. C., Huszar, G., (2010), Double probing individual human spermatozoa: aniline blue staining for persistent histones and fluorescence in situ hybridization for aneuploidies, *Fertil Steril,* 93(7),. 2255-2261.

[63] Ozmen, B., Koutlaki, N., Youssry, M., Diedrich, K., Al-Hasani, S. (2007), DNA damage of human spermatozoa in assisted reproduction: origins, diagnosis, impact and safety, *Reprod BioMed Online,* 14(3), 384-395.

[64] Parrella, A., Keating, D., Cheung, S., Xie, P., Stewart, J. D., Rosenwaks, Z., Palermo, G. D., (2019), A treatment approach for couples with disrupted sperm dna integrity and recurrent ART failure, *J Assist Reprod Genet,* 36(10), 2057-2066.

[65] Paul, C., Melton, W., Saunders, T. K. (2008), Do heat and deficits in DNA repair pathways have a negative impact on male infertility, *MHR-Basic Sci Reprod Med,* 14(1), 1-8.

[66] Perry, A. C. F., Wakayama, T., Kishikawa, H., Kasai, T., Okabe, M., Toyoda, Y., Ryuzo, Y., (1999), Mammalian transgenesis by intracytoplasmic sperm injection, *Science,* 284(5417), 1180-1183.

[67] Quin, M. M., Jalalian, L., Riberio, S., Ona, K., Demirci, U., Cedars, M. I., Rosen, M. P., (2018), Microfluidic sorting selects sperm for clinical use with reduced DNA damage compared to density gradient centrifugation with swim-up split semen samples, *Human Reprod,* 33(8), 1388-1393.

[68] Ragheb, A. M., Ibrahim, R. M., Elbatanouny, A. M., Moussa, A. S., Abdelbary, A. M., Sayed, O. M., Elbadawy, M. S., Shaker, H. A. Hamdi, S. O. (2018), Role of sequential semen samples in infertile men candidates for assisted reproduction: a prospective study, *African J Urol,* 24, 363-367.

[69] Ramlau-Hansen, C. H., Toft, G., Jensen, M. S., Strandberg-Larsen, K., Hansen, M. L., Olsen, J., (2010), Maternal alcohol consumption during pregnancy and semen quality in the male offspring: two decades of follow-up', *Human Reprod,* 25(9), 2340-2345.

[70] Ravnborg, T. L., Jensen, T. K., Andersson, A., Toppari, J., Skakkebaek, N. E., Jorgensen, N., 2011, 'Prenatal and adult exposures to smoking are associated with adverse effects on reproductive hormones, semen quality, final height and body mass index', *Human Reprod,* 26(5), 1000-1011.

[71] Richthoff, J., Spano, M., Giwercman, Y .L., Frohm, B., Jepson, K., Malm, J., Elzanaty, S., Stridsberg, M. Giwercman, A. 2002, The impact of testicular and accessory sex gland function on sperm chromatin integrity as assessed by the sperm chromatin structure assay (SCSA)', *Human Reprod,* 17(12), 3162-3169.

[72] Sakkas, D., Alvarez, J. G., (2010), Sperm DNA fragmentation: mechanisms of origin, impact on reproductive outcome, and analysis, *Fertil Steril,* 93(4), 1027-1036.

[73] Sallam H. N., Farrag A., Agameya A. F. A., El-Garem Y., Ezzeldin F. 2005. The use of the modified hypo-osmotic swelling test for the selection of immotile testicular spermatozoa in patients treated with ICSI: a randomized controlled study. *Human Reprod*; 20(12):3435–3440.

[74] Santi D., Giorgia S., Simoni M., (2018), Sperm DNA fragmentation index as a promising predictive toll for male infertility diagnosis and treatment management – meta-anaylses', *Reproduct BioMed Online,* 37(3), 315-326.

[75] Sharpe, R. M. (2010), Enviromental/lifestyle effects on spermatogenesis, *Phil Trans Royal Soc,* 365, 1697-1712, doi: 10.1098/rstb.2009.0206.

[76] Shen, Z., Shi, B., Wang, T., Jiao, J., Shang, X., Wu, Q., Zhou, Y., Cao, T., Du, Q., Wang, X., Li, D., (2019), Characterization of the sperm proteome and reproductive outcomes with in vitro, fertilization after a reduction in male ejaculatory abstinence period, *Mol Cell Proteomics,* 18, 109-117.

[77] Simoes, R., Feitosa, W. B., Mendes, C. M., Marques, M. G., Nicacio, A. C., De Barros, F. R. O., Visintin, J. A. Assumpcao, M. E. O. A., (2009), Use of chromomycin a3 staining in bovine sperm cells for detection of protamine deficiency', *Biotechnic Histochem,* 84(3), 79-83.

[78] Simon, L., Castillo, J., Oliva, R., Lewis, E. M. (2011), Relationships between human sperm protamines, DNA damage and assisted reproduction outcomes, *Reprod Biomed Online,* 23, 724-734.

[79] Sivanaryana, T., Krishna, C. R., Parkash, G. J., Krishna, K. M., Madan, K., Rani, B. S., Sudhakar, G., Raju, A. R. (2012), Casa derived human sperm abnormalities: correlation with chromatin packing and DNA fragmentation, *J Assist Reprod Genet,* 29, 327-1334.

[80] Stanger J. D., Long V., John L., Yovich J. L. Almahbobi G. 2010. Hypo-osmotic swelling test identifies individual spermatozoa with minimal DNA fragmentation, *Reprod BioMed Online;* 21(4):474-484

[81] Tan, J., Taskin, O., Albert, A. Bedaiwy, M. A., (2019), Association between sperm DNA fragmentation and idiopathic recurrent pregnancy loss: a systematic review and a meta-analysis', *Reprod BioMed Online,* 38(6), 951-960.

[82] Taylor S. L., Yoon S. Y., Morshedi M. S., Lacey D. R., Jellerette T., Fissore R. A., Oehninger S. Complete globozoospermia associated with PLCζ deficiency treated with calcium ionophore

and ICSI results in pregnancy. *Reprod Biomed Online.* 2010 Apr; 20(4):559-564.

[83] Tesarik, J., Tesarik, R. M. Mendoza, C., (2006), Sperm nuclear DNA damage: update on the mechanism, diagnosis and treatment, *Reprod BioMed Online,* 12(6), 715-721.

[84] Varshini. J., Srinag, B. S., Kalthur, G., Krishnamurthy, H., Kumar, P., Rao, S. B. S. Adiga, S. K., (2011), OOR sperm quality and advancing age are associated with increased sperm DNA damage in infertile men', *Andrologia,* 44, 642-649.

[85] Venkatesh, S., Singh, A., Shamsi, M. B., Thilagavathi, J., Kumar, R., Mitra, D. K. Dada, R. (2011), Clinical significance of sperm dna damage threshold value in the assessment of male infertility, *Reprod Sci,* 18(10), 1005-1013.

[86] Wignera, S. L. Vita, R. (2018), Thyroid dysfunction and semen quality', *Internat J Immunopathol Pharmacol,* 32, 1-5.

[87] Ward, W. S. (2011), Regulating DNA supercoiling: sperm points the way, *Biol Reprod,* 84, 841-843.

[88] Westerlakan, L. V. D., Naaktgeboren, N., Verburg, H., Dieben, S., Helmerhorst, F. M., (2006), Conventional in vitro fertilization versus intracytoplamic sperm injection in patients with borderline semen: a randomized study using sibling oocytes, *Fertil Steril,* 85(2), 395-400.

[89] Xi, Q., Zhang, Z., Wang, R., Li, L., Li, L., Zhu, H., Liu, R. Luo, L., (2019), Obstetric and perinatal outcomes of intracytoplasmic sperm injection for infertile men with Y chromosome microdeletions, *Medicine,* 98(41), e17407.

[90] Zorn, B., Golob, B., Ihan, A., Kopitar, A., Kolbezen, M., (2012), Apoptotic sperm biomarkers and their correlation with conventional sperm parameters and male fertility potential, *J Assist Reprod Genetics,* 29, 357-364.

In: Intracytoplasmic Sperm Injection (ICSI) ISBN: 978-1-53619-762-4
Editor: Murid Javed

Chapter 3

The Effects of Sperm Quality on Embryo Development after Intracytoplasmic Sperm Injection; Impact of Sperm on Embryo Quality and Treatment Outcome

Yousef Al Helou[1], Salman Ali Aldakhilallah[2], Naif Hamdan Alharbi[2], Nafisa Ali[3] and Jaffar Ali[4,*]

[1]Fakih IVF Dubai, United Arab Emirates
[2]Department of Reproductive Endocrine and Infertility Medicine, King Fahad Medical City Riyadh, Saudi Arabia
[3]Androcryogenics (M) Sdn Bhd, Shah Alam, Malaysia
[4]Department of IVF Maternity and Children Hospital, Dammam, Kingdom of Saudi Arabia

* Corresponding Author's E-mail: jaffarali.abdullah@gmail.com.

ABSTRACT

This chapter explains indications for ICSI, characteristics of a normal sperm, the process of normal fertilization, embryo development, genetic/epigenetic sperm abnormalities, and effects of abnormal sperm on embryo development. Initially ICSI was indicated for severe male factor infertility or after failed IVF; however, its indications have expanded with some labs exclusively performing ICSI.

Keywords: ICSI indications, normal sperm, sperm abnormality, embryo development, chromosomal abnormality in sperm

INTRODUCTION

The first live-born baby after conventional *in vitro* fertilization (IVF) was reported in 1978 (Steptoe, 1978). Despite the success of IVF in many clinics across the globe, it was overwhelmed with poor fertilization and fertilization failure despite the presence of sufficient number of oocytes. These cases with low fertilization or lack of fertilization were correlated to couples where the male partner had poor semen parameters (Cohen, 1984, Mahadevan, 1984). The advent of intracytoplasmic sperm injection (ICSI) is considered a revolutionary achievement in the field of assisted reproductive technology (ART) (Palermo, 2014) as ICSI has been utilized to largely resolve almost all of male fertility issues.

The ICSI overcame fertilization failure faced by conventional IVF (Pereira, 2016), resulting in birth of millions of babies to parents that would otherwise remain childless. It is well evident that ICSI technique is able to fertilize most of the mature oocytes regardless of sperm features (Palermo, 1993; 1995, Palermo and Neri, 2014). In this chapter, the effects of sperm quality on embryo development after ICSI are reviewed.

Indications for ICSI

Initially, ICSI was used to treat patients with male-factor infertility where the semen included one or more abnormal parameters that are assumed to be responsible for fertilization failure in conventional IVF (Palermo 1995; Palermo and Kocent, 2014). Presence of high level of anti-sperm antibodies in semen could result in fertilization failure during conventional IVF (Cline and Kutteh, 2009) for which ICSI is applied to circumvent fertilization failure. Subsequently, ICSI was used to treat patients with obstructive azoospermia (Schlegel and Palermo, 1995, Schlegel and Cohen, 1995) and non-obstructive azoospermia in patients that demanded surgical extraction of sperm (Palermo and Goldstein, 1999; Palermo and Schlegel, 1999). It has been utilized in patients with Klinefelter's syndrome (Palermo and Schlegel, 1998), patients with anejaculation due to paraplegia or any other cause (Chung et al., 1998), and even in azoospermia after chemotherapy (Chan et al., 2001). ICSI is used in patients who do not have mature sperm and round spermatid injection (ROSI; Tanaka et al., 2015), round spermatid nuclear injection (ROSNI; Hannay, 1995), elongated spermatid injection (ELSI; Tesarik and Mendoza, 1996) or secondary spermatocyte injection (SECSI; Sofikitis et al., 1998) has to be performed.

The non-male factor indications of ICSI include poor quality oocytes (Alikani et al., 1995), low oocyte yield (Moreno et al., 1998), prior fertilization failure with conventional IVF (Roest et al., 1998) and injection on day one after failed IVF on day zero (Morton et al., 1997), in cases requiring PGT (Thornhill et al., 2005), after *in vitro* maturation (IVM) (Hwang et al., 29), for fertilizing cryopreserved oocytes (Gook and Edgar, 2007) and HIV and hepatitis C discordant couple (Savasi et al., 2013).

Spermatogenesis

Spermatogenesis is the entire sequence of events that lead to the formation of mature sperm. In the immature testes, germ line stem cells (spermatogonia) are located at the basement membrane of the seminiferous tubules. At puberty, spermatogonia start to produce haploid spermatozoa. Spermatogonia are divided into three types based on morphological and functional properties: Type A dark (Adark), Type A pale (Apale), and Type B spermatogonia. Adark spermatogonia are the regenerative reserve of the testis. Apale spermatogonia show a comparably high mitotic activity and make up the functional reserve (Neto et al., 2016). Type B spermatogonia mark the entry of differentiation and meiosis (Sharpe, 2006). During puberty, Adark spermatogonia are mitotically active and occupy the stem cell niches within the seminiferous tubules of the testis. The Figure 1 (A) provides an overview of the male urogenital system and the Figure 1 (B) shows spermatogentic components. In contrast, this stem cell population shows low mitotic activity in the adult testis and serves as the stem cell reserve, which is only activated upon damage of the germ cell epithelium. Meiosis starts with the differentiation of B spermatogonia into preleptotene primary spermatocytes. Following meiosis, spermiogenesis begins. This process involves morphological transformations including the formation of an acrosome and a flagellum. The formation of a typical sperm head requires condensation of chromatin, elongation of the nucleus, and the removal of cytoplasm (Sharpe, 2006).

Characteristics of Normal Sperm

Assessment of sperm morphology is associated with a number of difficulties related to lack of objectivity, variation in interpretation or poor performance in external quality-control assessments. The method recommended by WHO is a simple normal/abnormal classification, with optional tallying of the location of abnormalities in abnormal spermatozoa (WHO, 2010).

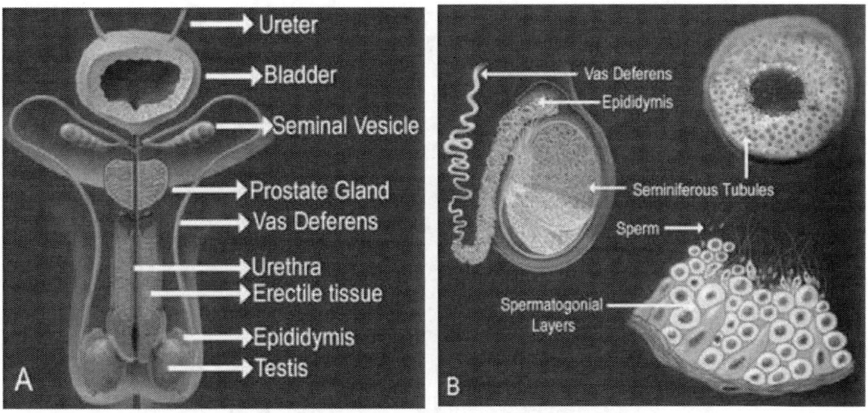

Figure 1. (A) Different components of male urogenital system. The sperm are formed in the testes, stored in the epididymis and transported via vas deferens to the urethra for ejaculation. The secretions from seminal vesicles and prostate glands make bulk of the ejaculatory volume. The urine and semen share the same urethra. (B) A diagram showing histological components involved in spermatogenesis. The sperm are formed from the spermatogonial cells in seminiferous tubules. The rounded immotile cells are transformed into sperm which gains the ability to move because of a flagellum. See Figure 2 for typical structure of a sperm.

Spermatozoa consist of a head, neck, middle piece (midpiece), principal piece and endpiece. As the endpiece is difficult to see with a light microscope, the cell can be considered to comprise a head (and neck) and tail (midpiece and principal piece). For a spermatozoon to be considered normal, both its head and tail must be normal (Figure 2). All borderline forms should be considered abnormal.

The head should be smooth, regularly contoured and generally oval in shape. The length of the head is 4.0 to 5.0 μM and the width should be 2.5 to 3.5 μM. There should be a well-defined acrosomal region comprising 40–70% of the head area (Mortimer and Menkveld, 2001; Alhelou, 2017). The acrosomal region should contain no large vacuoles, and not more than two small vacuoles, which should not occupy more than 20% of the sperm head. The post-acrosomal region should not contain any vacuoles.

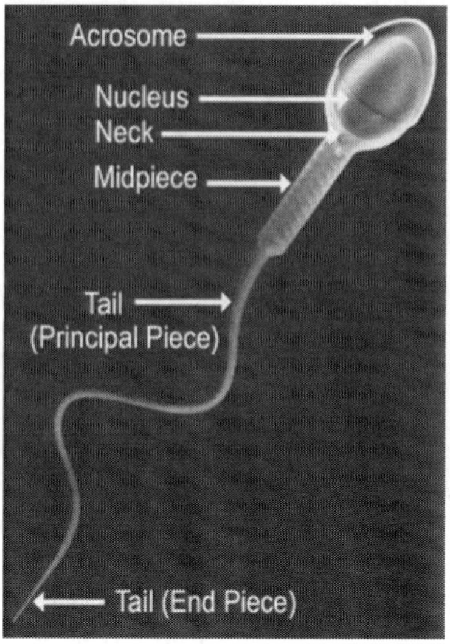

Figure 2. A diagrammatic explanation of various components of a normal sperm.

Head defects are large or small head, tapered, pyriform, round, amorphous, vacuolated (more than two vacuoles or >20% of the head area occupied by unstained vacuolar areas), vacuoles in the post-acrosomal region, small or large acrosomal areas (<40% or >70% of the head area), double heads, or any combination of these.

The midpiece should be slender, regular and should measure 2.0 – 2.5 μM in length and less than 1 μM in width. The major axis of the midpiece should be aligned with the major axis of the sperm head. Residual cytoplasm is considered an anomaly only when in excess, i.e., when it exceeds one third of the sperm head size (Mortimer and Menkveld, 2001).

Neck and midpiece defects are asymmetrical insertion of the midpiece into the head, thick or irregular, sharply bent, abnormally thin, or any combination of these.

Excess residual cytoplasm (ERC) is an anomaly that is associated with abnormal spermatozoa produced from a defective spermatogenic process. Spermatozoa characterized by large amounts of irregular stained cytoplasm, one third or more of the sperm head size, often associated with defective mid-pieces (Menkveld et al., 2001) are abnormal. This abnormal excess cytoplasm should not be called a cytoplasmic droplet (Mortimer and Menkveld, 2001; Grow et al., 1994).

The principal piece should have a uniform calibre along its length, be thinner than the midpiece, and be approximately 45 μM long (about 10 times the head length). It may be looped back on itself provided there is no sharp angle indicative of a flagellar break.

Principal piece defects include short, multiple, broken, smooth hairpin bends, sharply angulated bends, of irregular width, coiled, or any combination of these (WHO, 2010; Menkveld et al., 2001). The reference value for normal morphology is presence of ≥4% normal spermatozoa in the ejaculate.

The Natural Fertilization and Embryo Development Process

A step in the sperm function is termed capacitation which consists of alteration in the acrosome to prepare it to release the enzymes that will enable the sperm to pass through the granulosa cells, zona pellucida and the egg membrane. It occurs in the female reproductive tract as a result of contact with the fallopian tubes secretions (Bruc and Zernicka-Goetz, 2010).

When a capacitated sperm reaches the zona pellucida, it binds to a glycoprotein called ZP3. This binding results in a process called the acrosome reaction which releases enzymes that allows the sperm to drill the zona pellucida and reach the oocyte cell membrane and fuse with it. The fusion of the two membranes leads to formation of calcium waves and release of cortical granules; as a consequence the zona becomes impenetrable by other sperm (Rossant and Tam, 2009). After fusion the oocytes resumes meiosis and protrudes the second polar body and form the zygote which contains the male and female pronuclei.

The pronuclei disappear in preparation for division. The mitotic division starts by producing two blastomeres on the first day and continues to form six to 10 blastomeres in the third day. On the fourth day the blastomeres compact together to form the morula stage. On the fifth day, the size of the embryo increases and form the outer cells called the trophoblast and the inner cells mass which is called the embryoblast (Moore and Persaud, 2008).

GENETIC AND EPIGENETIC SPERM ABNORMALITY

The human ejaculate contains morphologically normal and abnormal spermatozoa. The abnormality may be in head, acrosome, midpiece, tail or combination of more than one abnormality. These can be detected under the microscope. However, the abnormality could be in the nucleus of the sperm. It has been reported that sperm of infertile men with teratozoospermia has abnormal numerical chromosomal makeup which is three times higher than the chromosomal abnormality in men with normal semen parameters (Harkonen et al., 2001, Calogero et al., 2001, Hristova et al., 2002).

Certain sperm morphological abnormalities are associated with chromosomal abnormality. Large head sperm show correlation with aneuploidy and polyploidy (Benzacken et al., 2001). Pin head sperm, double tail and nucleated head are associated with aneuploidy (Bernardini et al., 1998). Sperm head vacuoles are negatively correlated to fertilization, implantation and pregnancy (Braga et al., 2011).

Another sperm abnormality is the sperm DNA fragmentation. Some morphologically and chromosomally normal sperm exhibit sperm nucleus DNA damage that causes male infertility (Larson et al., 2000). It has been shown that sperm with damaged DNA can affect embryo cleavage by causing slow fragmentation and lowered blastocyst development (Seli et al., 2004, Virro et al., 2004).

Epigenetics is an additional level of data that complements the information in the genomic DNA sequence; it is considered as a marking system that regulates gene expression and hence the phenotype of the cell. An epigenetic mark is a chemical modification of the DNA bases that leads to a modification in chromatin structure. The mechanisms leading to epigenetic imprinting include DNA methylation, histone modification and RNA transcriptional mechanisms. DNA methylation is stable but reprogrammable, heritable, and affects the regulation of gene expression.

Human sperm obtain epigenetic information at the time of gametogenesis, such epigenetic information is organized through the preimplantation time. The epigenetic information of the egg and the sperm combine together at the time of fertilization, then get regulated and continue throughout the preimplantation period where gene expression is controlled. Therefore, any epigenetic abnormality in sperm affects the resulting embryos and offspring (Trasler, 2006). It has been shown that DNA methylation and histone methylation in zygotes obtained by ROSI has demonstrated differences as compared to ICSI which suggests epigenetic abnormality of the immature male gametes (Kishigami et al., 2006). Additionally, abnormal presence of methylated chromatin in the male pronucleus has been discovered in zygotes after ROSI (Yamazaki et al., 2007).

Moderate and severe oligozoospermic patients have incomplete methylation that occur at the H19 DMR gene in spermatozoa (Marques et al., 2004). Abnormal expression of genes PEG1, KCNQ1OT1, ZAC, PEG3 and SNRPN in sperm from infertile men specially in patients with moderate to severe oligospermia. Patients with impaired spermatogenesis showed abnormality in DNMT1 protein and mRNA expression (Omisanjo et al., 2007).

CHROMATIN ABNORMALITY

Sperm DNA fragmentation is considered as a type of abnormality that cannot be seen in the routine semen analysis. Sperm with damaged and fragmented DNA show inverse correlation with male fertility.

Sperm with fragmented DNA have the ability to fertilize oocytes at the same rate as by the DNA intact sperm and there is no correlation between sperm morphology and DNA integrity. It was shown that damaged sperm DNA affects embryonic cleavage negatively (Seli 2004). Sperm with fragmented DNA form embryos that exhibit slow cleavage and reduced blastocyst formation (Virro et al., 2004).

High prevalence of spontaneous pregnancy loss resulted from fragmented DNA sperm. Male patients with more than 30% fragmented DNA have high rate of multinucleated embryos after ICSI in contrast to patients with low fragmented DNA sperm (Zini et al., 2005). Multinucleated human embryos are correlated with reduced implantation and pregnancy rates.

Sperm with vacuoles have high incidence of damaged DNA. The vacuolated sperm have shown negative correlation with fertilization, implantation and pregnancy (Braga et al., 2011). Therefore, selection of sperm without vacuoles and other abnormalities for ICSI would enhance outcome (Bartoov et al., 2002).

Sperm Preparation

The sperm preparation in the ART lab aims to separate the motile and morphologically normal sperm from the seminal plasma (Baker et al., 1999) as the seminal plasma contains decapacitation factors and other cells that can cause sperm damage (Aitken et al., 1998). The use of density gradient and swim-up techniques can separate good quality sperm (Ng et al., 1992). The density gradient technique provides a safe method to prepare samples of virus-infected males (Savasi et al., 2007). Other preparation techniques for immotile sperm include exposing the sperm to pentoxifylline (Shen et al., 1991) and hypo-osmotic swelling test (Jeyendran and Zaneveld, 1986; Casper et al., 1996).

Sperm Selection for ICSI

To achieve the best results after ICSI, the embryologists tend to choose morphologically normal or borderline sperm for ICSI. However, certain sperm head defects are not visible during the ICSI procedure and this leads to poor results after ICSI. Such subtle defects are linked to poor pregnancy (Bartoov et al., 2002). This led some workers to the use of the technique of motile sperm organelle morphology examination (MSOME) which uses digital magnification at 6000x to select sperm without defects. It has been reported that sperm selected by MSOME have also led to reduced DNA fragmentation (Berkovitz et al., 2005). Performing ICSI using MSOME is termed as intracytoplasmic morphologically selected sperm injection (IMSI). The IMSI is helpful to patients with oligoasthenoteratozoospermia as this technique yielded higher pregnancy rate and less miscarriage rate (Antinori et al., 2008). However meta analyses and Cochrane reviews by various groups to determine usefulness of IMSI has provided conflicting results, some not in favour of IMSI (Duran-Retamal et al., 2020; Texeira et al., 2013), others showed low quality evidence in favour of IMSI (He et al., 2018; Texeira et al., 2020) and others with good outcome (Setti et al., 2014; 2010). It is obvious, that more conclusive evidence is required to determine usefulness of IMSI.

Another technique to select mature sperm with low DNA fragmentation is the use of hyaluronic acid (HA). Only mature sperm express HA receptors on the sperm head and have the ability to bind to the zona pellucida. Sperm that bind to solid state HA have less chromosomal abnormality (Jakab et al., 2005) and less DNA fragmentation (Cayli et al., 2004). Significant improvement in fertilization rate was achieved using sperm selected by HA technique (Nasr-Esfahani et al., 2008).

ICSI Process and Embryo Culture

The early attempts to achieve fertilization by injecting sperm into eggs were reported in 1962 for sea urchin (Hiramoto 1962) and in 1996 for mouse (Lin 1966). For the sake of historical accuracy, the first attempt to inject the human sperm into the human oocyte was reported in 1990 by Ng, then working at the National University of Singapore (Ng et al., 1990). He called the technique "MIMIC" (Micro-Insemination Micro-Injection into Cytoplasm) but this technique was not practiced in most countries due to regulation and the experimental nature of the technique until it was revisited a few years later by Palermo (Palermo et al., 1993). It is noteworthy that Ng was also the pioneer of the SUZI technique (Ng et al., 1991). The early trials to inject human sperm into human eggs faced high degeneration rate and low implantation rates (Lanzendorf et al., 1998). The earliest report of human ICSI from Europe was performed by Palermo (Palermo 1993) supposedly accidently during a SUZI procedure, as reported by Pereira (Pereira et al., 2016). This accidental fertilization of the human oocyte by the injection of sperm directly into the oocyte received considerable publicity worldwide that resulted in the universal adoption of this technique of insemination of ICSI as a novel approach in overcoming male infertility. This "accident" paved the way for the subsequent application of ICSI for the use in all types of spermatozoa regardless of their features.

Equipment required for ICSI are the inverted microscope with contrast objectives, two micromanipulators, one holding pipette and its holder and a micro injection pipette and its holder (Figure 3). All procedural steps in ICSI are performed under aseptic conditions and at physiological temperature. The ICSI petri dish contains drops of HEPES buffered medium and PVP covered with oil. The selected sperm is immobilized in the PVP medium and then injected using an injection pipette into the egg held in position using a holding pipette within a HEPES droplet. At the time of injection, the polar body is oriented at the 12 or 6 o'clock position and the sperm injected through at the 3 o'clock position.

After sperm injection, the oocytes are transferred into culture media and incubated under stable temperature, gases, humidity and pH untill the time of embryo transfer or freezing. The obstetric outcomes of ICSI pregnancies were similar to the outcomes of the pregnancies conceived with IVF and other ART methods (Wisanto et al., 1995).

Morphological Abnormality and Embryo Development

There is a noticeable reduction in fertilization rate in couples when the male partner suffered from abnormal sperm morphology (Terriou et al., 1997). Other reports showed direct relation between abnormal sperm morphology and poor embryo development and poor embryo quality (Parinaud et al., 1993). In addition there is a link between abnormal sperm morphology and delayed fertilization (Ron-El et al., 1991) and rate of embryo development (Salumets et al., 2002)

Globozoospermia is a known morphological abnormality with prevalence of 0.1% of infertile men (Dam et al., 2007).

Globozoospermic patients have sperm with round head that do not have acrosomal cap. Globozoospermia results from abnormal elongation of sperm head and acrosome formation during spermiogenesis (Zeyneloglu et al., 2002). Globozoospermia was linked to microdeletion in the AZFa and AZFb regions of the Y chromosome (Zeyneloglu et al., 2002).

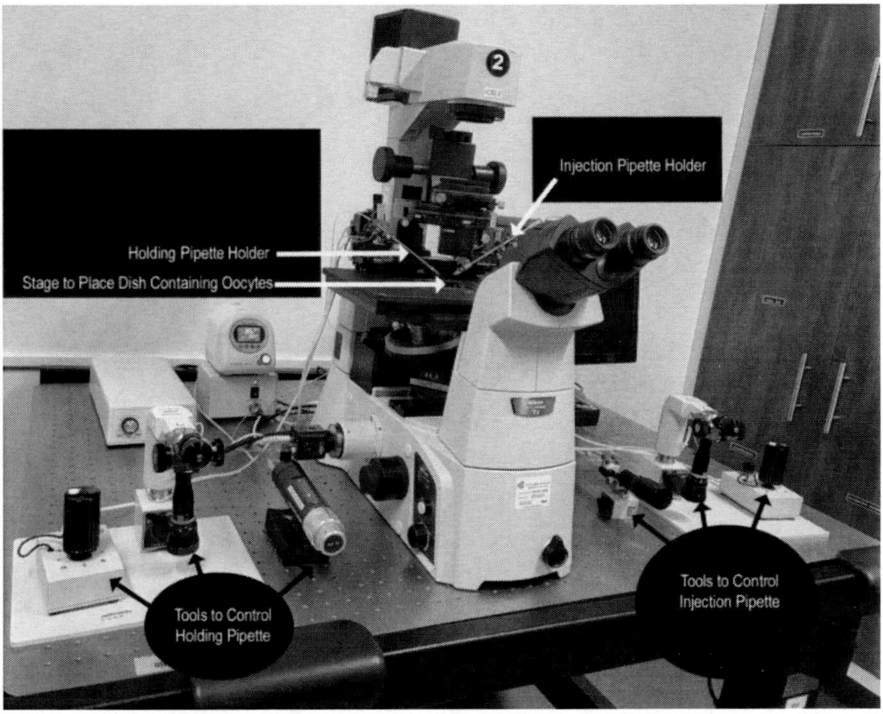

Figure 3. A picture of a typical ICSI set up showing all required components. Microscope and micromanipulation tools may very depending on the manufacturer of the equipment.

In conventional IVF globozoospermic patients have complete fertilization failure due to the disturbance of the zona pellucida penetration by sperm because of the absence of the acrosome. At the ICSI level there is poor fertilization of less than 40% (Trokoudes et al., 1995). Oocyte activation with calcium ionophore helps to increase the fertilization rate after ICSI with globozoospermic sperm (Dirican et al., 2008).

The lack of fertilization in globozoospermic patients is attributed to premature chromosome condensation of sperm (Schmiady et al., 2005), caused by protamine deficiency in the gloobozoospermic sperm head (Deemeh et al., 2007). Globozoospermia has been linked to increased prevalence of chromosomes aneuploidy (Carrell et al., 1999). Globozoospermia may have genetic origin as it occurs in siblings (Florke-Gerloff et al., 1984).

Effect of Abnormal Sperm on Embryo Morphokinetics

The advent of time-lapse incubators facilitated the continuous monitoring of the progress of embryos in culture and keep them under stable incubation conditions without the need to take the embryo outside the incubator for evaluation and this protects the embryo from environmental insults due to changes in temperature, pH and oxygen changes (Milewski and Ajduk, 2017; Alhelou et al., 2017; Alhelou et al., 2018,). The time-lapse incubator takes images of the embryo every few minutes and channels the images to make a video, which gives details on embryo quality, the timing of embryonic developmental events and the duration of such developmental events (Milewski et al., 2015).

Sperm tail abnormality was associated negatively with the early developmental stages until 4-cell stage. There is delay in the appearance or development of the pronuclei (PN) and its subsequent fading or disappearance, and in the development to the 3-cell or 4-cell stages. The mid-piece abnormality causes aberrations in the development of embryo from the 5-cell to the 9-cell stage. Finally, sperm head abnormality is associated negatively with development of the embryo from the 9-cell through the hatching blastocyst stages (Nikolova et al., 2020).

Conclusion

Sperm Morphology has an impact on the resulting embryo, implantation and live birth. This impact is observed clearly when using morphologically abnormal sperm. Morphologically abnormal sperm is associated with higher incidence of genetic, epigenetic and DNA fragmentation than morphologically normal sperm. The ICSI resolved fertilization issues associated with oligoasthenoteratozoospermia, but has had limited success with globozoospermia and immature sperm. The prognostic value of morphologically normal sperm remains debatable as there is inconsistent correlation between the morphology of the apparently normal sperm and its chromosomal content and chromatin integrity. The sperm selection techniques like IMSI and HA binding can offer somewhat better pregnancy rate and lower miscarriage rate for certain groups of patients but does not benefit all patient groups.

References

[1] Aitken, R., Gordon, E., Harkiss, D., Twigg, J., Milne, P., Jennings, Z. & Irvine D. S. (1998). Relative impact of oxidative stress on the functional competence and genomic integrity of human spermatozoa. *Biol Reprod*, *59*, 1037–1046.

[2] Alhelou, Y. (2017). Modern Evaluation of Sperm: Clinical application of the 5th Edition WHO manual for processing and Examining Semen in Allahbadia, G., Chawla, M., Das, R., Gandhi, G., Garcia, E., Merchant, R., Editors. The Art and Science of Assisted Reproductive Techniques (ART). *Jaypee publishers*, p. 268-273.

[3] Alhelou, Y., Mat Adenan, N. A. & Ali, J. (2018). Embryo culture conditions are significantly improved during uninterrupted incubation: A randomized controlled trial. *Reprod Biol*, *18*(1), 40-45.

[4] Alhelou, Y., Mat Adenan, N. A. & Ali, J. (2017). Embryo culture conditions are superior during uninterrupted incubation –

randomized controlled trial. *Reprod Biomed Online*, *35*(S1), E2-E3.

[5] Alikani, M., Palermo, G., Adler, A., Bertoli, M., Blake, M. & Cohen, J. (1995). Intracytoplasmic sperm injection in dysmorphic human oocytes. *Zygote*, *3*(4), 283–288.

[6] Antinori, M., Licata, E., Dani, G., Cerusico, F., Versaci, C., d'Angelo, D. & Antinori, S. (2008). Intracytoplasmic morphologically selected sperm injection: a prospective randomized trial. *Reprod Biomed Online.*, *16*, 835–841.

[7] Baker, G., Liu, D. Y. & Bourne, H. (1999). Assessment of the male and preparation of sperm for ARTs. In: Trounson, A.O., Gardner, D.K., Eds. *Handbook of In Vitro Fertilisation*. Boca Raton: CRC Press, 99-126.

[8] Bartoov, B., Berkovitz, A., Eltes, F., Kogosowski, A., Menezo, Y. & Barak, Y. (2002). Real-time fine morphology of motile human sperm cells is associated with IVF-ICSI outcome. *J Androl*, *23*, 1–8.

[9] Benzacken, B., Gavelle, F., Martin-Pont, B., Dupuy, O., Lievre, N., Hugues, J. & Wolf, J. (2001). Familial sperm polyploidy induced by genetic spermatogenesis failure: case report. *Hum Reprod*, *16*, 2646–2651.

[10] Berkovitz, A., Eltes, F., Yaari, S., Katz, N., Barr, I., Fisman, A. & Bartoov, B. (2005). The morphological normalcy of the sperm nucleus and pregnancy rate of intracytoplasmic injection with morphologically selected sperm. *Hum Reprod*, *20*, 185–190.

[11] Bernardini, L., Borini, A., Preti, S., Conte, N., Flamigni, C., Capitanio, G. & Venturini, P. (1998). Study of aneuploidy in normal and abnormal germ cells from semen of fertile and infertile men. *Hum Reprod*, *13*, 3406–3413.

[12] Braga, D., Setti, A., Figueira, R., Nichi, M., Martinhago, C., Iaconelli, A. & Borges, Jr. E. (2011). Sperm organelle morphologic abnormalities: contributing factors and effects on intracytoplasmic sperm injection cycles outcomes. *Urology*, *78*, 786–791.

[13] Bruc, A. & Zernicka-Goetz, M. (2010). Developmental control of the early mammalian embryo: competition among heterogeneous cells that biases cell fate. *Curr Opin Genet Dev*, *20*, 485–491.

[14] Calogero, A., De Palma, A., Grazioso, C., Barone, N., Romeo, R., Rappazzo, G. & D'Agata, R. (2001). Aneuploidy rate in spermatozoa of selected men with abnormal semen parameters. *Hum Reprod*, *16*, 1172–1179.

[15] Carrell, D., Emery, B. & Liu, L. (1999). Characterization of aneuploidy rates, protamine levels, ultrastructure, and functional ability of round-headed sperm from two siblings and implications for intracytoplasmic sperm injection. *Fertil Steril.*, *71*, 511–516.

[16] Casper, R., Meriano, J., Jarvi, K., Cowan, L. & Lucato, M. L. (1996). The hypoosmotic swelling test for selection of viable sperm for intracytoplasmic sperm injection in men with complete asthenozoospermia. *Fertil Steril.*, *65*, 972–976.

[17] Cayli, S., Sakkas, D., Vigue, L., Demir, R. & Huszar, G. (2004). Cellular maturity and apoptosis in human sperm: creatine kinase, caspase-3 and Bclx expression in mature and diminished maturity spermatozoa. *Mol Hum Reprod*, *10*, 365–372.

[18] Chan, P., Palermo, G., Veeck, L., Rosenwaks, Z. & Schlegel, P. (2001). Testicular sperm extraction combined with intracytoplasmic sperm injection in the treatment of men with persistent azoospermia postchemotherapy. *Cancer*, *92*(6), 1632–1637.

[19] Chung, P. H., Palermo, G., Schlegel, P. N., Veeck, L. L., Eid, J. F. & Rosenwaks, Z. (1998). The use of intracytoplasmic sperm injection with electroejaculates from anejaculatory men. *Hum Reprod*, *13*(7), 1854–1858.

[20] Cohen, J., Edwards, R., Fehilly, C., Fishel, S., Hewitt, J., Rowland, G., Steptoe, P. & Webster, J. (1984). Treatment of male infertility by *in vitro* fertilization: factors affecting fertilization and pregnancy. *Acta Eur Fertil*, *15*(6), 455–465.

[21] Cline, A. M. & Kutteh, W. H. (2009). Is there a role of autoimmunity in implantation failure after *in-vitro* fertilization? *Curr. Opin. Obstet. Gynecol.*, *21*, 291–295.

[22] Dam, A., Feenstra, I., Westphal, J., Ramos, L., van Golde, R. & Kremer, J. (2007). Globozoospermia revisited. *Hum Reprod Update.*, *13*, 63–75.

[23] Deemeh, M., Tavalee, M., Razavi, S. & Esfahani, M. (2007). Evaluation of protamine deficiency and DNA fragmentation in two globozoospermia patients undergoing ICSI. *Iran J Fertil Steril*, *1*, 85–88.

[24] Dirican, E., Sik, A., Vicdan, K., Sozen, E. & Suludere, Z. (2008). Clinical pregnancies and live births achieved by intracytoplasmic injection of round headed acrosomeless spermatozoa with and without oocyte activation in familial globozoospermia: a case report. *Asian J Androl.*, *10*, 332–336.

[25] Duran-Retamal, M., Morris, G., Achilli, C, Gaunt, M., Theodorou, E., Wael Saab, W., Serhal, P. & Seshadri, S. (2020). Live birth and miscarriage rate following intracytoplasmic morphologically selected sperm injection vs intracytoplasmic sperm injection: An updated systematic review and meta-analysis. *Acta Obstet Gynecol Scand*, *99*(1), 24-33.

[26] Florke-Gerloff, S., Topfer-Peterson, E., Muller-Estrel, W., Mansouri, A., Schatz, R. & Schirre, C. (1984). Biochemical and genetic investigation of round-headed spermatozoa in infertile men including two brothers and their father. *Andrologia*, *16*, 187–202.

[27] Gook, D. & Edgar, D. (2007). Human oocyte cryopreservation. *Hum Reprod Update*, *13*, 591–605.

[28] Grow, D., Oehninger, S., Seltman, H., Toner, J., Swanson, R., Kruger, T. & Muasher, S. (1994). Sperm morphology as diagnosed by strict criteria: probing the impact of teratozoospermia on fertilization rate and pregnancy outcome in a large *in vitro* fertilization population. *Fertil Steril*, *62*, 559–567.

[29] Hannay, T. (1995). New Japanese Ivf Method Finally Made Available in Japan. *Nat Med.*, *1*(4), 289-290.

[30] Harkonen, K., Suominen, J. & Lahdetie, J. (2001). Aneuploidy in spermatozoa of infertile men with teratozoospermia. *Int J Androl*, *24*, 197–205.

[31] He, F., Mei-Jiao Wang, M. J., Li, S. L., Zhang, C. Y., Li-Na. & Hu, L. N. (2018). *IMSI versus ICSI for male factor infertility: A meta-analysis. Zhonghua Nan Ke Xue*, *24*(3), 254-262.

[32] Hiramoto, Y. (1962). Microinjection of the live spermatozoa into sea urchin eggs. *Exp Cell Res.*, *27*, 416–426.

[33] Hristova, R., Ko, E., Greene, C., Rademaker, A., Chernos, J. & Martin, R. (2002). Chromosome abnormalities in sperm from infertile men with asthenoteratozoospermia. *Biol Reprod*, *66*, 1781–1783.

[34] Hwang, J., Lin, Y. & Tsai, Y. (2000). *In vitro* maturation and fertilization of immature oocytes: a comparative study of fertilization techniques. *J Assist Reprod Genet*, *17*, 39–43.

[35] Jakab, A., Sakkas, D., Delpoano, E., Cayli, S., Kovanci, E., Ward, D., Revelli, A. & Huszar, G. (2005). Intracytoplasmic sperm injection: a novel selection method for sperm with normal frequency of chromosomal aneuploidies. *Fertil Steril*, *84*, 1665–1673.

[36] Jeyendran, R. S. & Zaneveld, L. J. D. (1986). Human sperm hypoosmotic swelling test. *Fertil Steril*, *46*, 151-152.

[37] Kishigami, S., Van Thuan, N., Hikichi, T., Ohta, H., Wakayama, S., Mizutani, E. & Wakayama, T. (2006). Epigenetic abnormalities of the mouse paternal zygotic genome associated with microinsemination of round spermatids. *Dev Biol*, *289*, 195-205.

[38] Lanzendorf, S., Maloney, M., Veeck, L., Slusser, J., Hodgen, G. & Rosenwaks, Z. (1988). A preclinical evaluation of pronuclear formation by microinjection of human spermatozoa into human oocytes. *Fertil Steril.*, *49*(5), 835–842.

[39] Larson, K., DeJonge, C., Barnes, A., Jost, L. & Evenson, D. (2000). Sperm chromatin structure assay parameters as

predictor of failed pregnancy following assisted reproductive techniques. *Hum Reprod*, *15*, 1717–1722.

[40] Lin, T. (1966). Microinjection of mouse eggs. *Science.*, *151*(3708), 333–337.

[41] Mahadevan, M. & Trounson, A. O. (1984). The influence of seminal characteristics on the success rate of human *in vitro* fertilization. *Fertil Steril*, *42*(3), 400–405.

[42] Marques, C., Carvalho, F., Sousa, M. & Barros, A. (2004). Genomic imprinting in disruptive spermatogenesis. *Lancet*, *363*, 1700-1702.

[43] Menkveld, R., Wong, W., Lombard, C., Wetzels, A., Thomas, C., Merkus, H. & Steegers-Theunissen, R. (2001). Semen parameters, including WHO and strict criteria morphology, in a fertile and subfertile population: an effort towards standardization of *in-vivo* thresholds. *Hum Reprod*, *16*, 1165-1171.

[44] Milewski, R. & Ajduk, A. (2017). Time-lapse imaging of cleavage divisions in embryo quality assessment. *Reproduction.*, *154*, 37-53.

[45] Milewski, R., Kuc, P., Kuczynska, A, Stankiewicz, B., Lukaszuk, K. & Kuczynski, W. (2015). A predictive model for blastocyst formation based on morphokinetic parameters in time-lapse monitoring of embryo development. *J Assist Reprod Genet.*, *32*, 571-579.

[46] Moore, K. & Persaud, T. (2008). The beginning of human development: first week in Moore, K., Persaud, T. Editors. *The developing human.*, 14-39.

[47] Moreno, C., Ruiz, A., Simon, C., Pellicer, A. & Remohi, J. (1998). Intracytoplasmic sperm injection as a routine indication in low responder patients. *Hum Reprod*, *13*, 2126–2129.

[48] Mortimer, D. & Menkveld, R. (2001). Sperm morphology assessment—historical perspectives and current opinions. *J Andr*, *22*, 192-205.

[49] Morton, P., Yoder, C., Tucker, M., Wright, G., Brockman, W. & Kort, H. (1997). Reinsemination by intracytoplasmic sperm

injection of 1-day-old oocytes after complete conventional fertilization failure. *Fertil Steril*, *68*(3), 488–491.

[50] Nasr-Esfahani, M., Razavi, S., Vahdati, A., Fathi, F. & Tavalaee, M. (2008). Evaluation of sperm selection procedure based on hyaluronic acid binding ability on ICSI outcome. *J Assist Reprod Genet.*, *25*, 197–203.

[51] Neto, F., Bach, P., Najari, B., Li, P. & Goldstein, M. (2016). Spermatogenesis in humans and its affecting factors. *Semin Cell Dev Bio*, *59*, 10–26.

[52] Ng, F., Liu, D. & Baker, H. (1992). Comparison of Percoll, mini- Percoll and swim-up methods for sperm preparation from abnormal semen samples. *Hum Reprod*, *7*, 261–266.

[53] Ng, S. C., Bongso, T. A., Sathananthan, A. H. & Ratnam, S. S. (1990). Micro-manipulation: its relevance to human IVF. *Fertil. Steril.*, *53*, 203-219.

[54] Ng, S. C., Bongso, A. & Ratnam, S. S. (1991). Microinjection of human oocytes: a technique for severe oligoasthenoteratozoospermia. *Fertil Steril*, *56*(6), 1117-11123.

[55] Nikolova, S., Parvanov, D., Georgieva, V., Ivanova, I., Ganeva, R. & Stamenov, G. (2020). Impact of sperm characteristics on time-lapse embryo morphokinetic parameters and clinical outcome of conventional *in vitro* fertilization. *Andrology.*, *00*, 1–10.

[56] Omisanjo, O., Biermann, K., Hartmann, S., Heukamp, L., Sonnack, V., Hild, A., Brehm, R., Bergmann, M., Weidner, W. & Steger, K. (2007). DNMT1 and HDAC1 gene expression in impaired spermatogenesis and testicular cancer. *Histochem Cell Biol*, *127*, 175-181.

[57] Palermo, G. D., Cohen, J., Alikani, M., Adler, A. & Rosenwaks, Z. (1995). Intracytoplasmic sperm injection: a novel treatment for all forms of male factor infertility, *Fertil Steril*, *63*(6), 1231–1240.

[58] Palermo, G. D., Goldstein, M., Veeck, L. L., Rosenwaks, Z. & Schlegel, P. N. (1999). Testicular sperm extraction with

intracytoplasmic sperm injection for nonobstructive azoospermia: testicular histology can predict success of sperm retrieval. *J Urol*, *161*(1), 112–116.
[59] Palermo, G., Joris, H., Derde, M. P., Camus, M., Devroey, P. & Van Steirteghem, A. (1993). Sperm characteristics and outcome of human assisted fertilization by subzonal insemination and intracytoplasmic sperm injection. *Fertil Steril*, *59*(4), 826–835.
[60] Palermo, G., Kocent, J., Monahan, D., Neri, Q. & Rosenwaks, Z. (2014). Treatment of male infertility. Methods. *Mol Biol*, *1154*, 385–405.
[61] Palermo, G., Neri, Q., Schlegel, P. & Rosenwaks, Z. (2014). Intracytoplasmic sperm injection (ICSI) in extreme cases of male infertility. *PLoS On*, *9*(12), e113671.
[62] Palermo, G., Schlegel, P., Hariprashad, J., Ergün, B., Milienk, A., Zaninovic, N., Veeck, L. & Rosenwak, Z. (1999). Fertilization and pregnancy outcome with intracytoplasmic sperm injection for azoospermic men. *Hum Reprod*, *14*(3), 741–748.
[63] Palermo, G., Schlegel, P., Sills, E., Veeck, L., Zaninovic, N., Menedez, S. & Rosenwak, Z. (1998). Births after intracytoplasmic injection of sperm obtained by testicular extraction from men with nonmosaic Klinefelter's syndrome. *N Engl J Med*, *338*(9), 588–590.
[64] Parinaud, J., Mieusset, R., Vieitez, G., Labal, B. & Richoilley, G. (1993). Influence of sperm parameters on embryo quality. *Fertil Steril*, *60*, 888–892
[65] Pereira, N., Cozzubbo, T., Cheung, S. & Palermo, G. (2016). Lessons learned in andrology: from ntracytoplasmic sperm injection and beyond. *Andrology*, *4*(5), 757–760.
[66] Roest, J., Van Heusden, A. M., Zeilmaker, G. H. & Verhoeff, A. (1998). Treatment policy after poor fertilization in the first IVF cycle. *J Assist Reprod Genet*, *15*, 18–21.
[67] Ron-El, R., Nachum, H., Herman, A., Golan, A., Caspi, E. & Soffer, E. (1991). Delayed fertilization and poor embryonic

development associated with impaired semen quality. *Fertil Steril*, *55*, 338–344.

[68] Rossant, J. & Tam, P. (2009). Blastocyst lineage formation, early embryonic asymmetries and axis patterning in the mouse. *Development*, *136*, 701–713.

[69] Salumets, A., Suikkari, A., Molos, T., Soderstrom- Anttila, V. & Tuuri, T. (2002). Influence of oocytes and spermatozoa on early embryonic development. *Fertil Steril.*, *78*, 1082–1087.

[70] Savasi, V., Ferrazzi, E., Lanzani, C., Oneta, M., Parrilla, B. & Persico, T. (2007). Safety of sperm washing and ART outcome in 741 HIV-1-serodiscordant couples. *Hum Reprod*, *22*, 772–777.

[71] Savasi, V., Mandia, L., Laoreti, A. & Cetin, I. (2013). *Reproductive assistance in HIV serodiscordant couples Human Reproduction Update*, *19*(2), 136–150.

[72] Schlegel, P., Cohen, J., Goldstein, M., Gilbert, B., Palermo, G. & Rosenwak, Z. (1995). Cystic fibrosis gene mutations do not affect sperm function during *in vitro* fertilization with micromanipulation for men with bilateral congenital absence of vas deferens. *Fertil Steril*, *64*(2), 421–426.

[73] Schlegel, P., Palermo, G., Alikani, M., Alder, A., Reing, A. & Cohen, J. (1995). Micropuncture retrieval of epididymal sperm with *in vitro* fertilization: importance of *in vitro* micromanipulation techniques. *Urology*, *46*(2), 238–41.

[74] Schmiady, H., Schulze, W., Scheiber, I. & Pfuller, B. (2005). High rate of premature chromosome condensation in human oocytes following microinjection with round-headed sperm: case report. *Hum Reprod*, *20*, 1319–1323.

[75] Seli, E., Gardner, K., Schoolcraft, B., Moffatt, O. & Sakkas, D. (2004). Extent of nuclear DNA damage in ejaculated spermatozoa impacts on blastocyst development after *in vitro* fertilization. *Fertil Steril.*, *82*, 378–383.

[76] Setti, S. A., Ferreira, R. C., Paes de Almeida Ferreira Braga, D., de Cássia Sávio Figueira, R., Iaconelli, A. Jr. & Borges, E. Jr. (2010). Intracytoplasmic sperm injection outcome versus

intracytoplasmic morphologically selected sperm injection outcome: a meta-analysis. *Reprod Biomed Online*, *21*(4), 450-455.
[77] Setti, A. S., Braga, D. P., Figueira, R. C., Iaconelli, A. Jr. & Borges, E. (2014). Intracytoplasmic morphologically selected sperm injection results in improved clinical outcomes in couples with previous ICSI failures or male factor infertility: a meta-analysis. *Eur J Obstet Gynecol Reprod Biol.*, *183*, 96-103.
[78] Shen, M., Chiang, P., Yang, R., Hong, C. & Chen, S. (1991). Pentoxifylline stimulates human sperm motility both *in vitro* and after oral therapy. *Br J Clin Pharmacol.*, *31*(6), 711–714.
[79] Sofikitis, N., Mantzavinos, T., Loutradis, D., Yamamoto, Y., Tarlatzis, V. & Miyagawa, I. (1998). Ooplasmic injections of secondary spermatocytes for non-obstructive azoospermia. *Lancet*, *351*(9110), 1177-1178.
[80] Sharpe, R. (2006). Regulation of spermatogenesis. In: Knobil E, Neill J, editors. *The physiology of reproduction*. New York: Raven Press, 1363–1434.
[81] Steptoe, P. C. & Edwards, R. G. (1978). Birth after the reimplantation of a human embryo. *Lancet*, *2*(8085), 366.
[82] Tanaka, A., Nagayoshi, M., Takemoto, Y., Tanaka, I., Kusunoki, H., Watanabe, S., Kurodad, K., Takedad, S., Itoe, M. & Yanagimachi, R. (2015). Fourteen babies born after round spermatid injection into human oocytes. *Proc Natl Acad Sci*, *12*(47), 14629–14634.
[83] Terriou, P., Giorgetti, C., Auquier, P., Hans, E., Spach, J., Salzmann, J. & Roulier, R. (1997). Teratozoospermia influences fertilization rate *in vitro* but not embryo quality. *Hum Reprod,*, *12*, 1069–1072.
[84] Tesarik, J. & Mendoza, C. (1996). Spermatid injection into human oocytes. Laboratory techniques and special features of zygote development. *Hum Reprod*, *11*(4), 772-779.
[85] Teixeira, D. M., Barbosa, M. A. P., Ferriani, R. A., Navarro, P. A., Raine-Fenning, N., Nastri C. O., Wellington, P. & Martins,

W. P. (2013). Regular (ICSI) versus ultra-high magnification (IMSI) sperm selection for assisted reproduction. *Cochrane Database Syst Rev.*, *25*, (7), CD010167.

[86] Teixeira, D. M., Miyague, A. H., Mariana Ap Barbosa, A. A. P., Navarro, P. A., Raine-Fenning, N., Nastri, C. O. & Martins, W. P. (2020). Regular (ICSI) versus ultra-high magnification (IMSI) sperm selection for assisted reproduction. *Cochrane Database Syst Rev.*, *21*, 2(2), CD010167.

[87] Thornhill, A. R., deDie-Smulders, C. E., Geraedts, J. P., Harper, J. C., Harton, G. L., Moutou, C., Robinson, R., Schmuyzler, A., Skriven, P., Sermon, K. M. & Wilton, L. (2005). ESHRE PGD Consortium 'Best practice guidelines for clinical preimplantation genetic diagnosis (PGD) and preimplantation genetic screening (PGS)'. *Hum Reprod*, *20*, 35–48.

[88] Trasler, J. (2006). Gamete imprinting: setting epigenetic patterns for the next generation. *Reprod Fertil Dev*, *18*, 63-39.

[89] Trokoudes, K., Danos, N., Kalogirou, L., Vlachou, R., Lysiotis, T. & Georghiades, N. (1995). Pregnancy with spermatozoa from a globozoospermic man after intracytoplasmic sperm injection treatment. *Hum Reprod*, *10*, 880–882.

[90] Virro, M., Larson-Cook, K. & Evenson, D. (2004). Sperm chromatin structure assay (SCSA) parameters are related to fertilization, blastocyst development and ongoing pregnancy in *in vitro* fertilization and intracytoplasmic sperm injection cycle. *Fertil Steril*, *81*, 1289–1295.

[91] Wisanto, A., Magnus, M., Bonduelle, M., Camus, M., Tournaye, H., Liebaers, I., Steirteghem, A. & Devroey, P. (1995). Obstetric outcome of 424 pregnancies after intracytoplasmic sperm injection. *Hum Reprod*, *10*(10), 2713–2718.

[92] World Health Organization. (2010). *Laboratory Manual for the Examination of Human Semen and Sperm–Cervical Mucus Interaction.* 5th edn. Cambridge: Cambridge University Press.

[93] Yamazaki, T., Yamagata, K. & Baba, T. (2007). Time-lapse and retrospective analysis of DNA methylation in mouse preimplantation embryos by live cell imaging. *Dev Biol*, *304*, 409-419.

[94] Zeyneloglu, H., Baltaci, V., Duran, H., Erdemli, E. & Batioglu, S. (2002). Achievement of pregnancy in globozoospermia with Y chromosome microdeletion after ICSI. *Hum Reprod*, *17*, 1833–1836.

[95] Zini, A., Merian, J., Kader, K., Jarvi, K., Laskin, C. A. & Cadesky, K. (2005). Potential adverse effect of sperm DNA damage on embryo quality after ICSI. *Hum Reprod*, *12*, 3476–3480.

In: Intracytoplasmic Sperm Injection (ICSI) ISBN: 978-1-53619-762-4
Editor: Murid Javed

Chapter 4

INCREASING LINKS BETWEEN MALE FERTILITY AND DEFECTIVE OOCYTE ACTIVATION: AN EMERGING ROLE FOR PHOSPHOLIPASE C ZETA

***Junaid Kashir*[1,2,*] *and Serdar Coskun*[1,3]**
[1]Alfaisal University, College of Medicine, Riyadh, Saudi Arabia
[2]Department of Comparative Medicine, King Faisal Specialist Hospital & Research Center, Riyadh, Saudi Arabia
[3]Department of Pathology and Laboratory Medicine, King Faisal Specialist Hospital & Research Center, Riyadh, Saudi Arabia

ABSTRACT

Oocyte activation is a fundamental event at mammalian fertilization. In mammals, this process is initiated by a series of characteristic calcium (Ca^{2+}) oscillations, induced by a sperm-specific phospholipase C (PLC) termed PLCzeta (PLCζ). Dysfunction/reduction/deletion of PLCζ is associated with forms of male infertility where sperm is unable to initiate Ca^{2+} oscillations and oocyte activation, specifically in cases of fertilization failure.

* Corresponding Author's E-mail: jkashir@alfaisal.edu.

Defective PLCζ accompanied by abnormal patterns of Ca^{2+} release are increasingly suspected to underlie abnormal early embryogenesis. It also seems increasingly likely that cases of male infertility associated with poor efficacies of embryogenesis and recurrent implantation failure are linked to cases of PLCζ defection. Herein, we overview recent studies expanding clinical associations of PLCζ with the increasing types of male factor conditions, where sperm exhibits absent/reduced levels, and abnormal localization patterns of PLCζ within the sperm head. We also discuss mounting identifications of mutations in PLCζ, and how they affect functions of individual PLCζ domain structure, resulting in abrogation of activity or mechanism of action. Such cases could potentially strongly benefit from relevant therapeutic and diagnostic applications of PLCζ following focused research efforts.

Keywords: male fertility, defective oocyte activation, phospholipase C zeta, PLC zeta, globozoospermia

INTRODUCTION

In recent years, the global health community has experienced significant attention towards reproductive health (Cousens et al., 2011). A large contributory factor driving such attention are data highlighting the growing issue of global infertility, defined as the incapacity (Rutstein & Shah, 2004) to bear offspring following 1-2 years of regular unprotected intercourse. Infertility affects both men and women, albeit in different ways, throughout the world. Indeed, such is the issue that the World Health Organization (WHO, 2010) has classified infertility as a disease, affecting ~1 in every 7 couples. However, only a few comparative analyses examining the state of global infertility have been performed, likely due to a scarcity of consistent population-based studies (Mascarenhas et al., 2012).

Indeed, the observation of prevailing infertility heavily relies on the definition used (Gurunath et al., 2011; Irvine, 1998). Although reliable data on infertility prevalence in the world is scarce, estimates suggest that ~60-80 million couples (~8-12% of the global population) experience infertility in some form (Deyhoul et al., 2017; Kumar &

Singh, 2015; Rutstein & Shah, 2004). While various causative factors have been proposed for various forms of infertility, it is now widely accepted that male infertility is increasingly attributed as a major causative factor underlying infertility (Kashir et al., 2010). A suite of specialized laboratory techniques termed assisted reproductive technologies (ART) have yielded treatment options for affected couples, including *in vitro* fertilization (IVF) and intracytoplasmic sperm injection (ICSI). However, several conditions of severe male infertility remain untreatable even following ICSI (Botezatu et al., 2014). Treatment success currently collectively remain as low as 20-25% per cycle (Dyer, 2007; Ramadan et al., 2012), attributable to poor embryonic development or competency (Fauque et al., 2007; Pelinck et al., 2010), and poor sperm parameters (Loutradi et al., 2006). Indeed, selection of superior quality sperm improves embryogenic competency compared to without selection in the same infertile couples (Knez et al., 2011).

ICSI has developed as the default mode of treatment for couples with severe male factor infertility, as well as a number of non-male factor indications (Esteves et al., 2018; Knez et al., 2011). However, ~1-3% of ICSI cycles will fail, largely attributable to defective or failed fertilization (Amdani et al., 2016; Kashir et al., 2010; Mahutte & Arici, 2003; Sousa & Tesarik, 1994). Furthermore, however, specifically for cases of severe male factor infertility, ICSI is associated with lower rates of implantation and live birth rates compared to IVF (Boulet et al., 2015; Chambers et al., 2016; Esteves et al., 2018). A particular causative factor underlying this could potentially be recurrent implantation failure, driven by poor embryonic competency, which is understood to be a further factor underlying global infertility (Polanski et al., 2014).

Thus, sperm parameter quality, fertilization efficacy, and embryogenesis seem intricately linked. Indeed, sperm components involved at early fertilization may determine not just the efficacy of embryogenesis, but potentially the fate of the embryo itself. Herein, we discuss how components of a series of events, collectively termed oocyte activation, may serve a connecting role between various parameters of sperm fertility, the efficacy of subsequent embryogenesis, and potentially resultant ART success rates.

OOCYTE ACTIVATION, CALCIUM OSCILLATIONS, AND PHOSPHOLIPASE C ZETA

Oocyte activation is a series of concurrent and concerted fundamental events at fertilization in response to changes in concentrations of intracellular calcium (Ca^{2+}). Some vertebrates such as echinoderms, frogs, and fish exhibit a single Ca^{2+} wave in their eggs at fertilization, while mammalian (and several marine invertebrate) oocytes elicit a series of repetitive waves in distinct patterns, termed Ca^{2+} oscillations (Horner & Wolfner, 2008; Ito et al., 2011; Kashir et al., 2010; Kline & Kline, 1992; Miyazaki & Ito, 2006; Stricker, 1999; Swann & Ozil, 1994; Swann & Yu, 2008) (Figure 1), directly resulting from inositol trisphosphate (IP_3) generation (Amdani et al., 2016; Kashir et al., 2010; Miyazaki et al., 1993; Parrington, 2001; Parrington et al., 2007; Swann et al., 2006; Whitaker, 2006). These specific patterns of Ca^{2+}-release are inextricably connected to fertilization in all species studied thus far, and subsequent embryogenesis, in a species-specific manner (Brind et al., 2000; Ducibella et al., 2002; Ducibella et al., 2006; Fulton & Whittingham, 1978; Jellerette et al., 2000; Kashir et al., 2014; Kline & Kline, 1992; Miyazaki et al., 1993; Miyazaki et al., 1992; Swann & Yu, 2008; Xu et al., 2003).

Indeed, differential patterns of Ca^{2+} release altered protein expression profiles in early mouse embryos and rabbits, including rates of cell cycle progression and embryogenesis (Ducibella & Fissore, 2008; Ducibella et al., 2002; Ducibella et al., 2006; Malcuit et al., 2005; Miyazaki & Ito, 2006; Stitzel & Seydoux, 2007; Swann & Ozil, 1994), parameters that are now clinically considered as indicative of optimal embryogenesis and pregnancy success in humans (Wong et al., 2010; Yu et al., 2007).

Most evidence purports that the sperm delivers a specific soluble factor to the oocyte upon fertilization, which triggers Ca^{2+} release from intracellular stores (Coward et al., 2003; Coward et al., 2005; Dong et al., 2000; Kyozuka et al., 1998; Nakano, 1997; Stricker, 1997, 1999; Swann, 1990). A number of candidates have been proposed as this 'sperm factor' in what is known as the sperm factor hypothesis (Aarabi et al., 2009; Parrington et al., 1996; Sette et al., 1998; Sette et al., 2002; Wu et al., 2007). However, considering that the phosphoinositide signaling pathway is considered an essential component of oocyte activation, where intracellular IP_3 is generated by the hydrolysis of phosphatidylinositol 4,5-bisphosphate (PIP_2), binding to IP_3 receptors on the endoplasmic reticulum (ER) and causing Ca^{2+} release) (Aarabi et al., 2009; Ducibella et al., 2002; Ducibella et al., 2006; Fulton & Whittingham, 1978; Jones et al., 1995; Jones et al., 1998; Kashir et al., 2014; Kline & Kline, 1994; Miyazaki et al., 1993; Miyazaki et al., 1992; Nader et al., 2013; Swann, 1992), a potential phospholipase C (PLC) isoform had predominantly been suggested to be the elusive sperm factor. Puzzlingly, however, while numerous PLCs play distinct roles in both gametes during reproduction in mammals, such isoforms failed to elicit characteristic Ca^{2+} release upon injection into mouse oocytes (Coward et al., 2007; Igarashi et al., 2007; Kashir et al., 2014; Runft et al., 2004; Yin & Eckberg, 2009), indicating that these PLCs were not involved, at least in initiating, oocyte activation.

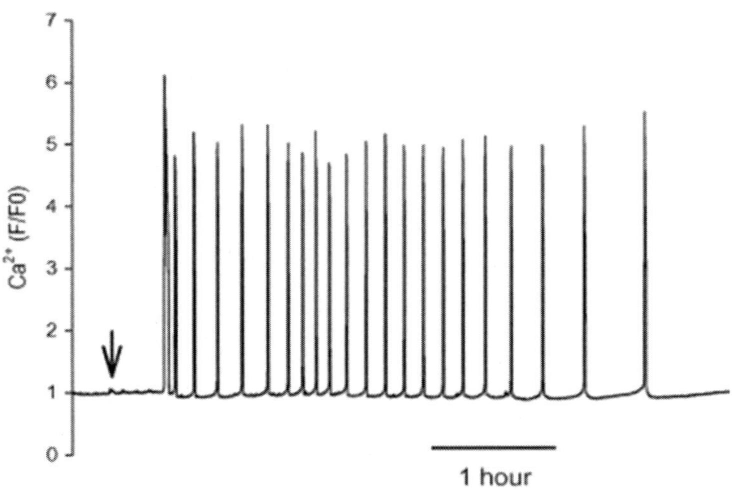

Figure 1. Representative recordings of intracellular Ca^{2+} release patterns. A mouse oocyte undergoing *in vitro* fertilization (IVF) using a Ca^{2+}-sensitive fluorescent dyes. The arrow indicates time of sperm addition to oocytes. Fluorescence is expressed as a ratio of the intensity divided by the starting fluorescence value. Figure adapted from Kashir et al., 2014 and Nomikos et al., 2013 with permission.

In 2002, a testis-specific PLC isozyme was identified, termed PLCzeta (PLCζ) (Cox et al., 2002; Saunders et al., 2002), which has since been characterized in multiple mammalian species (Bedford-Guaus et al., 2011; Bedford-Guaus et al., 2008; Cox et al., 2002; Yoneda et al., 2006; Yoon et al., 2008; Young et al., 2009). PLCζ exhibits characteristic X and Y catalytic domains forming the active site, a single C2 domain, and four tandem EF hand domains (Saunders et al., 2002; Suh et al., 2008). However, PLCζ uniquely lacks either a pleckstrin homology (PH), or Src homology (SH) domain, making PLCζ the smallest known mammalian PLC (~70kDa in humans; ~74kDa in mice) (73, 74). Native and recombinant PLCζ elicited Ca^{2+} oscillations similar to physiological patterns in both mouse and human oocytes, also supporting development to the blastocyst stage (Fujimoto et al., 2004; Kouchi et al., 2005; Kurokawa et al., 2005; Nomikos et al., 2005; Saunders et al., 2002) (Figure 2). Furthermore, diminishing PLCζ from sperm and sperm-extracts in turn abrogated Ca^{2+} release profiles in oocytes, significantly reducing litter sizes in mice (Bedford-Guaus et al., 2011; Coward et al., 2007; Coward et al., 2005; Coward et al., 2011; Cox et al., 2002; Ito et al., 2008; Knott et al., 2005; Saunders et al., 2002). Recent key studies that generated transgenic knockout (KO) mouse models where PLCζ was either abrogated or deleted concluded that PLCζ is the primary physiological stimulus of Ca^{2+} oscillations at fertilization, ensuring monospermy and effective oocyte activation and early embryonic development (Hachem et al., 2017; Nozawa et al., 2018).

PLCζ mRNA is first detectable at the spermatid stage in mice, with similar observations made in porcine, equine, and quail models (Kaewmala et al., 2011; Mizushima et al., 2009; Suh et al., 2008; Yin & Eckberg, 2009; Yoneda et al., 2006). PLCζ was suggested to be incorporated with the acrosome during the Golgi phase of human and mouse spermiogenesis (Aarabi et al., 2012). However, such observations have yet to be confirmed independently, and specific localization patterns throughout the various spermatogenic cells within testes require further elucidation. PLCζ localization in ejaculated/ mature sperm has been more extensively examined in mice, rats, hamsters, horses, pigs, bulls, and of course humans (Fujimoto et al.,

2004; Manandhar & Toshimori, 2003; Perry et al., 1999; Sutovsky et al., 2003; Young et al., 2009).

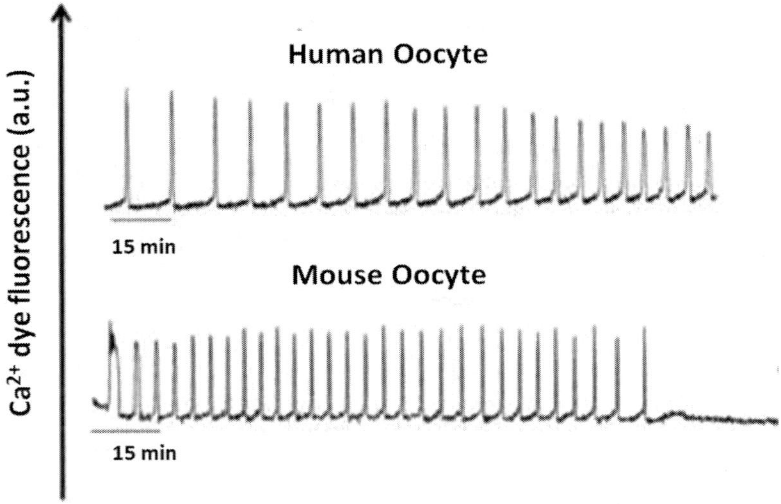

Figure 2. Representative recordings of intracellular Ca^{2+} release patterns. Human (top panel) and mouse (bottom panel) oocytes following microinjection of recombinant PLCζ. Fluorescence is expressed as a ratio of the intensity divided by the starting fluorescence value. Figure adapted from (Junaid Kashir et al., 2014)) and (Nomikos, Kashir, et al., 2013) with permission.

Immunofluorescence indicated PLCζ localization in mouse sperm to the post-acrosomal region; alongside a secondary acrosomal pattern (Fujimoto et al., 2004; Young et al., 2009). Populations of PLCζ have also been identified in acrosomal and post-acrosomal regions of porcine sperm, with an additional tail population (Kaewmala et al., 2011; Nakai et al., 2011). In equine sperm, PLCζ was found at the acrosomal and equatorial regions of the sperm head, alongside the principle piece of the flagellum (Bedford-Guaus et al., 2011). In humans, PLCζ was again identified in the acrosomal, equatorial, and post-acrosomal regions of the sperm head, alongside tail localizations (76, 97-101)(Grasa et al., 2008; Heytens et al., 2009; Kashir, Heynen, et al., 2011; Kashir, Jones, et al., 2011; Kashir et al., 2013; Yoon et al., 2008).

PLCζ localizations (Figure 3) seem dynamic within sperm, shifting from acrosomal/equatorial patterns to a dominantly post-acrosomal localization following capacitation in human, mouse/hamster, and bull sperm (Grasa et al., 2008; Mejía-Flores et al., 2017; Young et al., 2009). While equatorial PLCζ is considered to be perhaps the most physiologically relevant population to oocyte activation (postacrosomal in mice) allowing rapid diffusion of PLCζ into the oocyte at fertilization, acrosomal PLCζ populations have been proposed to also exert an as yet unknown role (Bi et al., 2009). Indeed, presence of equatorial PLCζ corresponded to intact acrosomes (Grasa et al., 2008; Heytens et al., 2009; Young et al., 2009), with PLCζ identified beneath the acrosomal cap in human sperm (Escoffier et al., 2015).

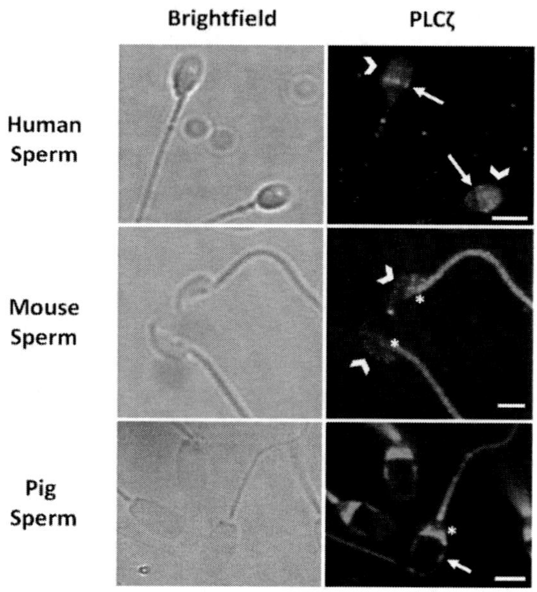

Figure 3. Representative immunofluorescence images indicating the localization patterns of sperm PLCζ in human (top panel), mouse (middle panel), and pig (bottom panel) sperm. PLCζ fluorescence is indicated in the right-most panels, and corresponding brightfield images are indicated in the left-most panels. White arrows indicate equatorial, white arrowheads indicate acrosomal, and white asterisks (*) indicate post-acrosomal localization patterns of PLCζ in the three species of sperm indicated. Images shown are indicative of predominant localization patterns observed throughout the published literature. White scale bars are indicative of 5μm.

Perhaps such differential localizations serve as multiple stores of PLCζ in sperm to ensure sufficient requisite levels are delivered to the oocyte for required patterns of Ca^{2+} release (Figure 4). Indeed, different species present species-specific physiological requirements in terms of PLCζ solubility and/or oocyte Ca^{2+} response (Kashir et al., 2014). Intriguingly, microinjection of equine tails into mouse oocytes resulted in high frequency Ca^{2+} oscillations, indicating presence of functional PLCζ (Bedford-Guaus et al., 2011).

Considering that eventually the entirety of the sperm is incorporated into the oocyte, including the midpiece and tail (Ramalho-Santos, 2011), such 'secondary' populations may temporally serve to ensure specific patterns of Ca^{2+} release. However, such specific assertions require further investigation, particularly within humans.

ICSI Failure and Oocyte Activation Deficiency

Given the significant success of ICSI, a complete failure of fertilization following ICSI is relatively rare (1–5% of cases). However, a characterizing feature of such failure is that this can happen regardless of sperm status, even using sperm with apparently normal parameters (Javed et al., 2011; Liu et al., 1995; Ludwig et al., 1999; Rubino et al., 2015; Sousa & Tesarik, 1994). Perhaps a larger issue associated with ICSI is not outright failure, but significantly lower or more moderate rates of fertilization success, remaining ≤ 30% in repeated ICSI cycles for some patients (Montag et al., 2012; Rubino et al., 2015). While the causative factor behind fertilization failure following conventional IVF is attributable to defects in sperm parameters which would prevent gamete fusion (morphology, concentration, motility), or even gamete expulsion, a failure of oocyte activation is attributed as the leading cause, if not the major contributory factor in all such cases alongside incorrect sperm injection, spindle defects, or premature sperm chromatin condensation (Rubino et al., 2015).

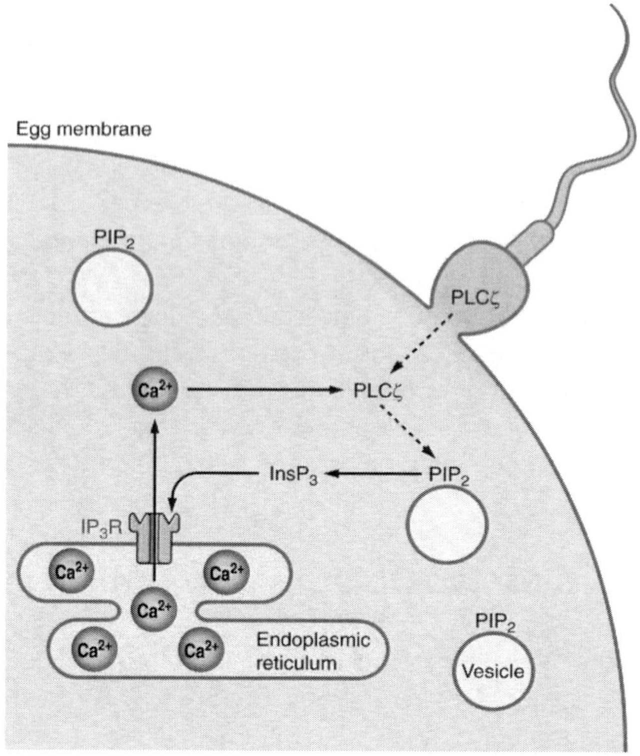

Figure 4. Schematic illustration of the proposed mechanism of PLCζ action. Following sperm andoocyte fusion the PLCζ diffuses into the oocyte and binds to cytoplasmic vesicular-PIP_2. The PIP_2 hydrolysis generates IP_3 which initiates Ca^{2+} release from the endoplasmic reticulum (ER). Increased cytosolic Ca^{2+} then further stimulates the activity of PLCζ, generating more IP_3. This positive feedback loop occurs throughout as PLCζ continues to diffuse across the ooplasm. This figure is adapted with permission from Swann & Lai (2016).

Thus, as it is an oocyte activation deficiency (OAD) that seems closely connected to ICSI failure, intricately associated components of oocyte activation such as PLCζ-induced Ca^{2+} release may underlie such cases of male infertility. Indeed, sperm of infertile men consistently exhibiting fertilization-failure following conventional IVF and/or ICSI were unable to elicit Ca^{2+} oscillations upon injection into mouse oocytes or produced severely abnormal patterns of Ca^{2+} release (Heytens et al., 2009; Yoon et al., 2008). Importantly, such sperm also exhibited absent/reduced levels and/or abnormal localization patterns of PLCζ within the sperm head (Heytens et al., 2009; Kashir, Jones, et al., 2011; Kashir et al., 2013; Yoon et al., 2008), suggesting that defective or abrogated PLCζ underlies such cases of fertilization failure (Kashir et al., 2010).

However, abnormal oocyte activation is not just limited to cases of fertilization failure, but also cases of successful fertilization, followed by abnormal or defective embryogenesis. Indeed, differential profiles of Ca^{2+} release altered profiles of gene expression at early embryogenesis (Ducibella et al., 2002; Ducibella et al., 2006), which in turn could also be altered by injection of differential levels of PLCζ in mammalian oocytes, resulting in differential frequencies and amplitudes of Ca^{2+} oscillations (Yamaguchi et al., 2017). Indeed, an ~4-fold range of effective PLCζ doses are able to result in successful activation and healthy development of blastocysts, which also corresponds to the same range of PLCζ levels observed in fertile human sperm (Kashir et al., 2013; Kashir et al., 2014; Yamaguchi et al., 2017).

Profiles of Ca^{2+} oscillations also determine healthy embryogenesis and successful transplantation rates in animal models, as well as cell cycle progression rates to the 2- and 4-cell stages of human oocytes, clinical indicators of normal embryogenesis and pregnancy success (Miyazaki & Ito, 2006; Swann & Ozil, 1994; Wong et al., 2010). Thus, Ca^{2+} oscillations at fertilization may not only be necessary for oocyte activation, but also of equal (if not more) importance for subsequent embryogenesis. Perhaps abnormalities in sperm PLCζ underlie not only infertility through fertilization failure, but also cases of male sub-fertility, whereby enough PLCζ may be delivered to oocytes to cause activation, but insufficient for embryonic competence. Indeed, ICSI is associated with lower rates of implantation and live birth compared to conventional IVF, with the Practice Committee of the American Society for Reproductive Medicine (ASRM) advising against the indiscriminate use of ICSI in non-male factor conditions of infertility (Chambers et al., 2016; Esteves et al., 2018; Kline & Kline, 1992; The Practice Committee, ASRM, 2012).

Defects in Phospholipase C Zeta and Conditions of Male Infertility

Unsurprisingly, most cases where ICSI application is mandatory (cases of severe male factor infertility) are now increasingly being associated with defective or abnormal profiles of PLCζ within the sperm head. Further to numerous mutations in PLCζ now identified in cases of both normal and abnormal sperm parameters, defective and/or abnormal expression and localization patterns of PLCζ have been observed in multiple male-specific conditions including abnormal sperm parameters and morphology (Azad et al., 2018a; Azad et al., 2018b; Escoffier et al., 2015; Janghorban-Laricheh et al., 2016; Kashir et al., 2010; Kashir et al., 2013; Tavalaee et al., 2018), sperm DNA fragmentation and oxidation (Park et al., 2015; Tavalaee et al., 2017a; Tavalaee et al., 2017b) and abnormal embryogenesis/pregnancies (Nikiforaki et al., 2014). Recent investigations (Kashir et al., 2020) using two antibodies with high specificity for PLCζ demonstrated that higher levels and specific localization patterns of PLCζ in human sperm correlated to optimal parameters of sperm fertility (motility, morphology, and semen volume), and increased fertilization success in a wider population of males undergoing fertility treatment. Such results indicated that PLCζ profiles are not only indicative of defective oocyte activation, but also perhaps general male fertility, and the efficacy of subsequent embryogenesis (Kashir, 2020).

PLCζ Domain Organization and Infertility Mutations

PLCζ is more potent in triggering Ca^{2+} oscillations within fertilizing oocytes compared to other PLCs (Nomikos et al., 2015a; Nomikos et al., 2015b; Nomikos et al., 2017). PLCζ domain structure, common to all PLC family members, consists of four tandem EF hand domains at the N-terminus, the catalytic X and Y domain in the center, followed by a single C-terminal C2 domain (Figure 5A). The X and Y catalytic domains are separated by the XY-linker (Kashir et al., 2010). The EF hands facilitate the high Ca^{2+} sensitivity of PLCζ, enabling maximal activity at resting Ca^{2+} levels within the oocyte prior to activation, while also assisting the XY-linker region with substrate targeting (Nomikos, Sanders, Parthimos, et al., 2015). The C2 domain is also essential for PLCζ function through PIP_2 targeting (Nomikos et al., 2005; Nomikos, Sanders, Parthimos, et al., 2015; Theodoridou et al., 2013). The XY-linker region of PLCζ shares ~60% sequence similarity to that of all PLCs and is responsible for PIP_2 targeting and attachments as well as hydrolysis through direct electrostatic interactions (Nomikos, Elgmati, Theodoridou, Calver, et al., 2011; Nomikos, Elgmati, Theodoridou, Georgilis, et al., 2011; Nomikos, Kashir, Swann, & Lai, 2013; Nomikos et al., 2007; Nomikos, Sanders, Parthimos, et al., 2015). All these succinct domains of PLCζ have now been associated with various mutations of PLCζ in cases of OAD and fertilization failure.

The first two PLCζ mutations identified were from the genomic DNA of an infertile male whose sperm, which while within normal parameters, exhibited repeated ICSI-failure. Both mutations were identified within the catalytic X and Y domains of PLCζ, disrupting local protein folding and reduction/abrogation of enzymatic activity (Heytens et al., 2009; Kashir, Heynen, et al., 2011; Kashir, Jones, et al., 2011; Kashir, Michalis Konstantinidis, Celine Jones, Bjorn Heindryckx, et al., 2012; Kashir, Michalis Konstantinidis, Celine Jones, Bernadette Lemmon, et al., 2012). Intriguingly, both mutations were heterozygous, with one mutation being inherited from the patient's father and the other from the patient's mother, implicating for the first time that maternally inherited loss-of-activity mutations could lead to male infertility (Junaid Kashir, Michalis Konstantinidis, Celine Jones, Bjorn Heindryckx, et al., 2012; Junaid Kashir, Michalis Konstantinidis, Celine Jones, Bernadette Lemmon, et al., 2012; Nomikos et al., 2017). Significantly, one of these two mutations (a Histidine to Leucine mutations at amino acid 233; H233L) was identified by a further two studies in separate cases (Ferrer-Vaquer, Barragan, Freour, Vernaeve, & Vassena, 2016; Torra-Massana et al., 2019), indicating that perhaps specific mutations could be common features within the human genome.

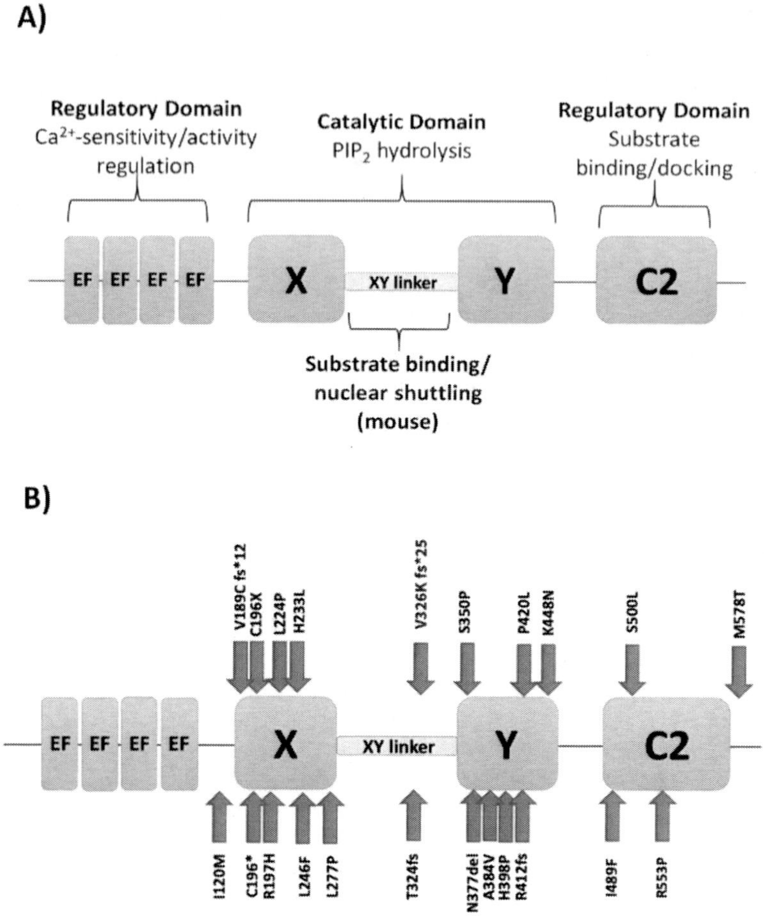

Figure 5. Schematic representation of PLCζ summarizing briefly **(A)** the functional roles of each domain group, and **(B)** indicating location of each mutation identified clinically thus far indicated by arrows. Each mutation is represented by the original amino acid, followed by the amino acid position number, and then the mutated amino acid.

Subsequently, a further homozygous mutation was reported from two infertile brothers, located at the C2 domain (Escoffier et al., 2016), which while exhibiting equivalent enzymatic activity to wild type PLCζ, displayed a dramatically reduced binding-affinity to PI(3)P and PI(5)P (Nomikos et al., 2017). Additionally, further studies have identified an additional 12 novel mutations, located throughout the EF-hands, the X and Y, XY-linker, and C2 domains. 10 of these were single nucleotide polymorphisms, altering the predicted local fold and diminishing the capacity for Ca^{2+} oscillations in mouse oocytes following corresponding cRNA injections (Dai et al., 2019; Ferrer-Vaquer et al., 2016; Mu et al., 2020; Torra-Massana et al., 2019). Two of these were frameshift variants, generating truncated proteins *in vitro* (Mu et al., 2020; Torra-Massana et al., 2019).

While further biochemical analyses are urgently required to ascertain whether these further variants of PLCζ are deleterious at physiological levels, needing accurate quantification in sperm and oocytes, all cases identified have in common reduced/absent levels of sperm PLCζ, and/or severely abnormal patterns of localization. Intriguingly, such observations of reduced mutated PLCζ levels can be correlated to *in vitro* studies whereby the first two identified mutations of PLCζ were over-expressed with a fluorescent tag in Human Embryonic Kidney 293-transformed (HEK293T) cells. Despite high transfection efficiency, mutant PLCζ isoforms exhibited a significantly lower level of fluorescence compared to WT, indicating perhaps lower levels of expression, and/or increased protein instability (Junaid Kashir, Jones, et al., 2011). Thus, it increasingly seems the case that deleterious PLCζ mutations are more widespread than previously thought, affecting activity and/or binding in the oocyte as well as potentially contributing towards decreased levels within sperm. Furthermore, single nucleotide polymorphisms (SNPs) have also been reported either within the PLCζ coding sequence or its associated bi-directional promoter in human patients (Ferrer-Vaquer et al., 2016; Yoon et al., 2008), as well as in bulls and horses (Pan et al., 2013; Schrimpf, Dierks, Martinsson, Sieme, & Distl, 2014) (Figure 5B).

SPERM ABNORMALITIES

Conventional semen analysis is currently the standard method to evaluate the severity of male infertility conditions, and whether to recommend use of ICSI. Sperm count, motility, and morphology are commonly used parameters assessed in this regard (Babayev, Park, & Bukulmez, 2014; Esteves et al., 2018; WHO, 2010). Indeed, ICSI was predominantly developed to tackle severe conditions of male factor infertility, before its current status of the most widely used method of ART (Esteves et al., 2018). Fertilization rates of sperm with abnormal parameters are significantly lower than normal parameters, with cumulative defects sequentially decreasing success rates (Nordhoff, Fricke, Schüring, Zitzmann, & Kliesch, 2015; Verza Jr & Esteves, 2008). Injection of morphologically abnormal sperm is associated with lower implantation rates (De Vos et al., 2003), while a higher incidence of meiotic errors in resultant embryos has been associated with lower sperm counts (Pang, 1999).

GLOBOZOOSPERMIA

The most studied example in relation to PLCζ and sperm parameters is that of globozoospermia, a condition characterized by round sperm heads devoid of an acrosome (Dam et al., 2006). Some patients present 100% morphologically abnormal sperm, while others exhibit mixed proportions (Escoffier et al., 2015). Regardless, patients with globozoospermia exhibit low success in oocyte activation without clinical intervention (De Braekeleer, Nguyen, Morel, & Perrin, 2015; Kashir et al., 2010), despite exhibiting in many cases normal sperm count and motility (Esteves et al., 2018). ICSI is usually the only treatment option in such cases, yet fertilization and pregnancy rates remain considerably low due to ineffective oocyte activation and embryo development (Esteves et al., 2018). Semen analysis of globozoospermic patients usually indicates sperm count and motility within normal parameters (Dam et al., 2006). Globozoospermia was regarded widely as untreatable until the introduction of ICSI (Lundin, Sjögren, Nilsson, & Hamberger, 1994; Palermo, 1992). However, fertilization rates are generally lower in patients with globozoospermia compared to patients with other indications following ICSI. Complete fertilization failure is observed in ~30% of globozoospermia cases (Chansel-Debordeaux, Dandieu, Bechoua, & Jimenez, 2015).

Several studies now strongly implicate three major genes; SPATA16, PICK1 and DPY19L2, as major genetic contributors towards etiologies of globozoospermia (Taylor et al., 2010). Proteomic analyses indicated differential expression of proteins involved in spermatogenesis, cytoskeletal processes, metabolism and motility, and acrosomal biogenesis (Sedo, Rawe, & Chemes, 2012; Liao, Xiang, Zhu, & Fan, 2009). A further characteristic of such sperm has repeatedly been demonstrated to be absent/reduced levels of PLCζ, alongside significantly altered profiles of localization in sperm (Aghajanpour et al., 2011; Kamali-Dolat Abadi, Tavalaee, Shahverdi, & Nasr-Esfahani, 2016; Kashir et al., 2010; J. Kashir et al., 2012; Taylor et al., 2010; Tejera et al., 2008). Intriguingly, when sperm from a globozoospermic population exhibiting an acrosomal bud were selected for ICSI, fertilization, embryogenesis, and pregnancy were successfully established. PLCζ localization in such sperm was at the acrosomal region, while PLCζ exhibited a dispersed pattern of localization in round headed sperm without an acrosomal bud that resulted in oocyte activation failure (Kamali-Dolat Abadi et al., 2016). A similar abnormal pattern of PLCζ localization was observed in a proposed mouse model of globozoospermia (Heytens et al., 2009), indicating that perhaps PLCζ profiles are strongly linked with specific morphological features of sperm.

Globozoospermia fertilization rates could be improved following the use of artificial methods of oocyte activation (assisted oocyte activation; AOA), such as Ca^{2+} ionophore treatment (Rybouchkin, Van der Straeten, Quatacker, De Sutter, & Dhont, 1997), suggesting that perhaps processes underlying sperm-based oocyte activation were defective. Indeed, treatment of globozoospermia with AOA nearly doubled fertilization and clinical pregnancy rates in ~72% of globozoospermic ICSI cycles. However complete fertilization failure still occurred in 6.3% of cycles, higher than the expected level observed in other cases of ICSI (1-3%) (Chansel-Debordeaux et al., 2015). Collectively, such data strongly suggest that more effective treatment protocols could be achieved perhaps including PLCζ as a universal AOA method to induce physiological Ca^{2+} oscillation patterns.

ABNORMAL SPERM PARAMETERS

Asthenozoospermia, characterized by reduced sperm motility, is a common contributor towards male infertility (Rybouchkin et al., 1997). Such reduction of sperm motility can be attributed to several factors, including as energy metabolism abnormalities, structural defects, and altered expression profiles of sperm motility proteins (Agarwal, Panner Selvam, & Baskaran, 2020; Cao et al., 2018; Kamali-Dolat Abadi et al., 2016; Martinez-Heredia, de Mateo, Vidal-Taboada, Ballesca, & Oliva, 2008; Rybouchkin et al., 1997; Saraswat et al., 2017; Sinha, Singh, Singh, & Yadav, 2019; Zhao et al., 2007). Proteomic analysis of sperm from asthenozoospermic patients also indicated differential expression patterns of the proteasome complex (Martinez-Heredia et al., 2008; Siva et al., 2010; Zhao et al., 2007), while differential expression was also observed in proteins associate with sperm function (Hashemitabar, Sabbagh, Orazizadeh, Ghadiri, & Bahmanzadeh, 2015), mitochondrial oxidative stress (Nowicka-Bauer et al., 2018), Ca^{2+} influx, and acrosomal acidification (Sinha et al., 2019). Similarly, in cases of Oligoasthenozoospermia, characterized by reduced sperm concentration and motility, proteomic characterization of seminal plasma implicated several proteins involved in oxidative stress (Herwig et al., 2013), binding and transporter activity, immunity, and hydrolase activity (Liu et al., 2018).

Indeed, recent studies now show that lower levels of PLCζ have been observed in teratozoospermic (Azad, Nazarian, Ghaffari Novin, Masteri Farahani, Piryaei, & Heidari, 2018), asthenoteratozoospermic (Park et al., 2015), and oligoasthenoteratozoospermic (Azad, Nazarian, Ghaffari Novin, Masteri Farahani, Piryaei, & Heidari, 2018; Azad, Nazarian, Ghaffari Novin, Masteri Farahani, Piryaei, Heidari, et al., 2018) patients, while a further negative correlation was present between PLCζ levels and cases of varicocele (Janghorban-Laricheh et al., 2016). Interestingly, in the case of asthenozoospermia, fertilization and blastocyst formation rates can reverted to comparably normal levels following co-injection of asthenozoospermic (non-viable) sperm with sperm extracts prepared from normal sperm, suggesting that such poor fertilization rates in these cases are attributable to the incapability of such sperm to activate oocytes (Ahmadi & Ng, 1999; Esteves et al.,

2018; Sermondade et al., 2011), i.e., PLCζ. Experiments increasing the proportion of non-viable human sperm by sonication followed by injection into mouse oocytes exhibited a decline of normal Ca^{2+} release patterns and embryogenesis rates (Hiroyuki Yazawa, Yanagida, Hayashi, & Sato, 2009).

AZOOSPERMIA

A further condition that could potentially be linked with defects in PLCζ is azoospermia, affecting ~10-15% of the infertile male population (Esteves, 2015). Characterized as either obstructive (blockage of the reproductive tract; OA) or nonobstructive (spermatogenic failure; NOA) azoospermia, the majority of azoospermic men are diagnosed with NOA (90-95%) (Tanaka et al., 2015). While microscopic testicular sperm extraction (micro-TESE) can be employed to extract testicular sperm for ICSI, ~30-40% of such patients do not exhibit testicular sperm or late-stage spermatids, presenting only round spermatids if at all (Tanaka et al., 2015).

While understandably few proteomic studies exist relating to azoospermia, studies performed in semen and testicular tissue of azoospermic patients have identified several potential biomarkers relating to spermatogenesis, spliceosome, cell cycle, proteasome, and energy metabolism (Bieniek, Drabovich, & Lo, 2016; Drabovich et al., 2013; Tanaka et al., 2015), all of which were differentially expressed in cases of azoospermia to varying degrees (Rybouchkin et al., 1997). Proteomic studies of cases involving NOA (such as varicocele), identified abnormalities in expression of heat shock proteins (HSPs), mitochondrial proteins, and cytoskeletal element (Chan, Sun, Shui, & Wu, 2013; Hosseinifar et al., 2013). Differential expression has also been reported of proteins involved in spermatogenesis, sperm maturation, motility, capacitation, acrosome reaction and fertilization success (Agarwal, Sharma, Durairajanayagam, Ayaz, et al., 2015; Agarwal, Sharma, Durairajanayagam, Cui, et al., 2015). Interestingly, these proteins were involved in processes including posttranslational modification, protein folding, ubiquitination, metabolism, mitochondrial dysfunction, enzyme regulation, and immunity (Agarwal, Sharma,

Durairajanayagam, Ayaz, et al., 2015; Agarwal, Sharma, Durairajanayagam, Cui, et al., 2015; Samanta et al., 2018).

To address such cases, round spermatid injection (ROSI) can be applied. Indeed, rodent ROSI resulted in successful fertilization and birth (Kimura & Yanagimachi, 1995; Ogura, Matsuda, & Yanagimachi, 1994; Tesarik & Mendoza, 1996; Yanagimachi et al., 2004). However, while ROSI has been successfully applied in humans (Barak et al., 1998; Gianaroli et al., 1999; Tesarik et al., 1996; Van den Veyver & Al-Hussaini, 2006; Vanderzwalmen et al., 1997), concerns surround he efficiency, safety, and practicality of such application (Ogonuki, Inoue, & Ogura, 2011; Ogura et al., 1994; Silber & Johnson, 1998; Silber, Johnson, Verheyen, & Van Steirteghem, 2000; Tanaka et al., 2018). Furthermore, rates of miscarriage following ROSI are quite high, ranging between 55-65% (Ogura et al., 1994; H. Yazawa, 2001). Mouse ROSI induced small profiles of Ca^{2+} oscillations (Kimura & Yanagimachi, 1995), indicating that round spermatids present with absent/reduced/deficient PLCζ. It is interesting that a structural criterion to identify round spermatids is the presence of an acrosomal vesicle/cap (Ogonuki et al., 2011; Ogura et al., 1994), a structure linked to presence of PLCζ, and fertilization and pregnancy success with globozoospermic sperm as previously discussed (Kashir et al., 2012; Sermondade et al., 2011).

In mouse, rabbit, rat, and pig, PLCζ protein has not been detected at the round spermatid stage (Aarabi et al., 2012; Bedford-Guaus et al., 2011; Kaewmala et al., 2011; Mizushima et al., 2009; Yoneda et al., 2006), while rat, mouse, and rabbit ROSI does not necessarily result in efficient oocyte activation without artificial induction, requiring additional stimuli to significantly increase success rates (Barratt et al., 2010; Hirabayashi, Kato, & Hochi, 2008; Hirabayashi et al., 2009; Loren & Lacham-Kaplan, 2006; Nicopoullos et al., 2019; Ogura et al., 1994; Yazawa, 2001; Yazawa et al., 2009). Perhaps it is the case that either insufficient or ineffective PLCζ is present at this stage. Similar investigations have yet to be performed on humans, but data suggest that human round spermatids contain at least some oocyte activating ability (Yazawa et al., 2009). Round spermatids from hamsters and humans are able successfully elicit Ca^{2+} oscillations following injection into mouse oocytes (Loren & Lacham-Kaplan, 2006; Hiroyuki Yazawa et al., 2009). However, this is likely due to increased activity of the human and hamster versions of the enzyme in mouse oocytes.

SPERM DNA FRAGMENTATION

Sperm nuclear status is another parameter gaining acceptance as a crucial consideration for successful ART outcomes, implicated in both embryogenic efficacy and pregnancy outcomes (Sedó et al., 2017; Nicopoullos et al., 2019). To this degree, testing of sperm DNA fragmentation (measuring proportions of sperm with damaged chromatin using specific probes or dyes) has emerged as potential prognostic indicator of male fertility (Esteves et al., 2018). Indeed, increased proportions of damaged or 'fragmented' sperm DNA (either single or double stranded breaks) are associated with poor sperm parameters, low fertilization and implantation rates, and increased miscarriage, regardless of ART method employed (Sedó et al., 2017; Lewis & Aitken, 2005; Nicopoullos et al., 2019; Osman, Alsomait, Seshadri, El-Toukhy, & Khalaf, 2015; Robinson et al., 2012; Virro, Larson-Cook, & Evenson, 2004). While the causes of DNA fragmentation have already been extensively studied and reviewed elsewhere (González-Marín, Gosálvez, & Roy, 2012; Rahimizadeh et al., 2019; Wright, Milne, & Leeson, 2014), studies are also now beginning to indicate negative correlations between decreased sperm PLCζ and increased DNA fragmentation and/or DNA oxidation (Gawecka et al., 2013; Park et al., 2015; Tavalaee, Kiani-Esfahani, et al., 2017; Tavalaee et al., 2017). However, such studies are significantly limited, both in scope and methodology employed (discussed later). Studies have not yet investigated whether specific motifs of PLCζ localization exhibit any relationship with sperm DNA fragmentation and/or other indicative factors.

While studies specifically studying potential relationships between PLCζ profiles and DNA fragmentation in sperm are relatively sparse, there is a relationship between the efficacy of oocyte activation and DNA damage repair in the oocyte. Sperm DNA damage cannot be repaired until the DNA becomes accessible by ooplasmic DNA repair pathways systems within the ooplasm (Rubino et al., 2015).

Furthermore, replication of the paternal pronuclei could be delayed in animal models, and embryo development arrested in cases of extensive DNA damage (Nicopoullos et al., 2019). Conversely, when DNA damage is less severe (such as in the case of single-stranded breaks), there is no detectable delay in cell cycle progression, but some level of DNA damage is detectable at subsequent mitosis (Gawecka, Ribas-Maynou, Benet, & Ward, 2015; Rubino et al., 2015).

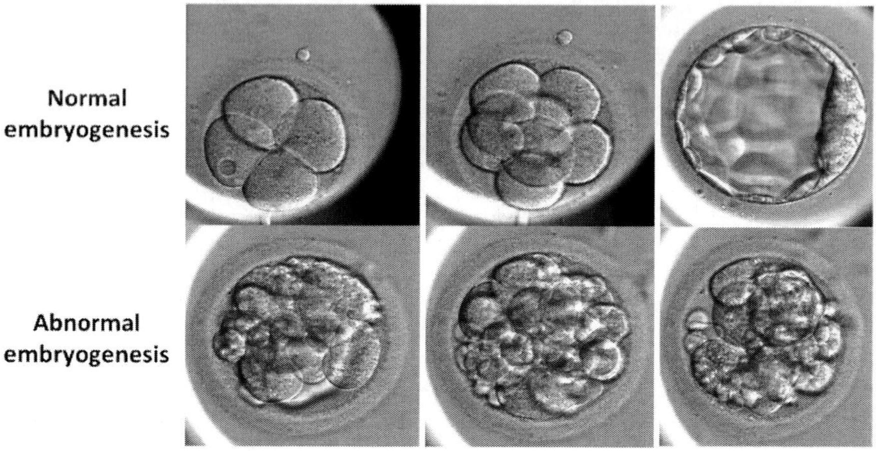

Figure 6. Representative time-lapse imaging of progressive stages (left to right) of normal (top panel) and abnormal (bottom panel) human embryogenesis. Images were taken during time-lapse assessment of embryo quality during fertility treatment.

Perhaps mechanisms exist within the oocyte to allow stalling of replication forks for DNA repair (Collins & Jones, 2016; Gawecka et al., 2015; Rubino et al., 2015). Indeed, while mechanisms of DNA damage repair in GV and MI oocytes is relatively well characterised (Martin, Bromfield, Aitken, Lord, & Nixon, 2018), the picture is less clear for MII oocytes immediately post-fertilization, although double stranded break DNA repair has recently been demonstrated to be mediated by non-homologous end-joining in mouse oocytes (Genescà et al., 1992). Rather intriguingly, studies have previously indicated that sperm DNA fragmentation, at least to a certain degree, can be repaired by the oocyte post-fertilization (Ahmadi & Ng, 1999; Desai et al., 2014), proposed to be dependent upon the balance between the amount/type of DNA damage and the individual oocytes DNA repair capacity (Martin et al., 2018). However, whether such pathways are related to PLCζ-induced oocyte activation is something that remains to be investigated.

Abnormal Embryogenesis

Current advancements in time lapse microscopy allow visualization of both nuclear and cytoplasmic dynamics during embryo culture, yielding continuous visualization and quantification of kinetic and morphological parameters (**Figure 6**). Such information allows predictive evaluation of embryo health and pregnancy success (Cruz et al., 2011; Pribenszky et al., 2010; Pribenszky, Nilselid, & Montag, 2017; Wong et al., 2010), correlating embryonic morphokinetic parameters as non-invasive biomarkers for embryo quality, blastocyst formation, and ultimately implantation, pregnancy and live birth (Cruz et al., 2011; Milewski, Szpila, & Ajduk, 2018; Pribenszky et al., 2017). Importantly, oocyte activation events accompanying fertilization, such as Ca^{2+} oscillations, are reflected by such morphokinetic parameters, particularly the 2nd and 3rd cell divisions post-fertilization, identified as the most potent predictive measurements (Santella & Dale, 2015). Particularly in humans, poor embryo quality can be correlated with too slow, or too fast, cell divisions (Cruz et al., 2011; Milewski et al., 2018; Parrington et al., 1996; Pribenszky et al., 2010; Pribenszky et al., 2017; Santella & Dale, 2015).

Nikiforaki et al., (2014) correlated abnormally reduced ability of sperm to induce Ca^{2+} release in mouse oocytes with defective embryogenesis in cases of hydatidiform moles; abnormal pregnancies associated with abnormal and/or absent embryogenesis. Human sperm leading to recurrent partial hydatidiform molar pregnancies could not elicit normal profiles of Ca^{2+} release following injection into both mouse and human oocytes, leading to OAD. This is particularly striking as human PLCζ is significantly more potent compared to mouse PLCζ in mouse oocytes (Ito et al., 2011), implying either a severely reduced level of PLCζ, or a severely diminished capacity for PIP_2 hydrolysis.

The temporal patterns of Ca^{2+} oscillations are species-specific in amplitude, duration, and frequency (Ducibella et al., 2002; Ducibella et al., 2006; Kashir et al., 2014; Miyazaki et al., 1993), the precise pattern of which seems to exert significant influence upon embryogenesis (Fulton & Whittingham, 1978; Kline & Kline, 1994; Miyazaki et al., 1992; Swann & Yu, 2008). Indeed, differential frequencies and amplitudes of Ca^{2+} altered protein expression profiles in embryos (Ducibella & Fissore, 2008; Ducibella et al., 2002; Ducibella et al., 2006), while specific patterns of Ca^{2+} release influenced cell-cycle progression, embryo compaction, blastocyst formation, and successful implantation of mammalian embryos (Ducibella et al., 2002; Ducibella et al., 2006; Miyazaki & Ito, 2006; Swann & Ozil, 1994). Thus, profiles of PLCζ-induced Ca^{2+} oscillations at fertilization may not only be necessary for oocyte activation, but also equally important for subsequent embryogenic events (Ducibella & Fissore, 2008; Wong et al., 2010; Yu et al., 2007), determining the efficacy of embryogenesis and potentially pregnancy success.

Therapeutic and Diagnostic Options for PLCz-Deficiencies

Collectively, increasing data necessitates the urgent investigation of PLCζ profiles in relation to various sperm parameters and conditions of male infertility that may not necessarily be directly linked to ICSI failure and OAD, but perhaps cases of successful fertilization, but poor embryogenesis and pregnancy rates (Figure 7). The occurrence of such increasing links between growing numbers of male fertility conditions and deficiencies in PLCζ indicates that PLCζ diagnostic and therapeutic options could be significant combative tools against general conditions of male infertility, and not just cases of ICSI-failure.

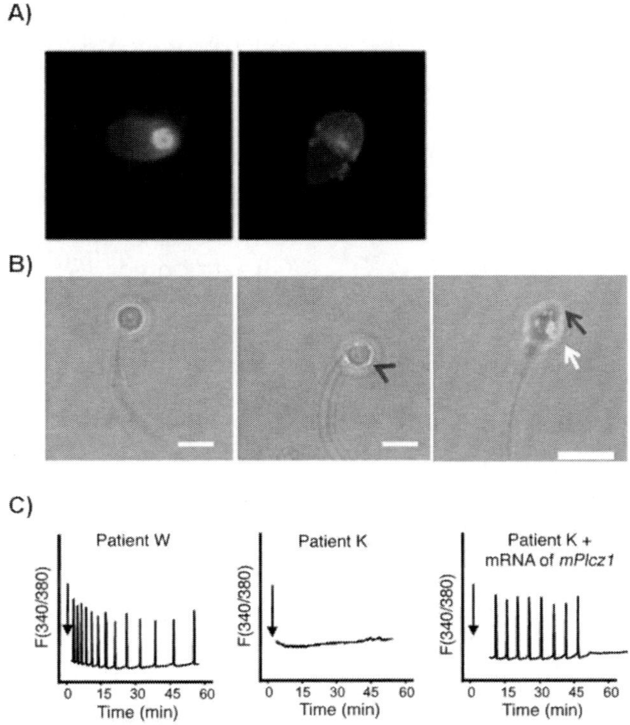

Figure 7. Representative immunofluorescence images of sperm indicating the associated profiles of PLCζ. **A)** Normozoospermic sperm where PLCζ is either absent (left panel) or exhibits abnormal punctate localisation (right panel). **B)** Globozoospermic sperm exhibits either absent or severely reduced levels of PLCζ, accompanied by abnormal localization (black arrowhead). However, in globozoospermic sperm exhibiting an acrosomal bud (black arrow), PLCζ is present at higher levels, albeit in abnormal localisation conformations (white arrow). **C)** Injection of normal human sperm in mouse oocytes exhibited normal Ca^{2+} oscillatory activity (left-most panel), while injection of sperm from an oocyte activation deficient male is unable to initiate Ca^{2+} release following microinjection in mouse oocytes (middle panel). However, injection of sperm from the same patient co-incident with mouse PLCζ mRNA successfully initiated fertilization-like Ca^{2+} oscillations. Figures adapted with permission from Kashir 2020).

Currently, defective oocyte activation can be clinically resolved through assisted oocyte activation (AOA), involving artificially mediated Ca^{2+} release through application of Ca^{2+} ionophores (Fawzy et al.,

2018; Norozi-Hafshejani, Tavalaee, & Nasr- Esfahani, 2019), significantly improving fertilization and implantation rates following ICSI (Murugesu et al., 2017). However, such methods induce a single Ca^{2+} transient, unlike the endogenous specific physiological pattern of Ca^{2+} oscillations observed during normal fertilization (Fawzy et al., 2018; Murugesu et al., 2017; Norozi-Hafshejani et al., 2019; Rogers et al., 2004). To this degree, PLCζ has long represented a physiologically endogenous alternative to AOA for treatment of ICSI failure and/or cases of OAD. Indeed, recombinant PLCζ is capable of inducing physiological patterns of Ca^{2+} oscillations in mouse and human oocytes (Nomikos, Yu, et al., 2013; Sanusi, Yu, Nomikos, Lai, & Swann, 2015) and is able to 'rescue' cases of OAD following co-injection of such sperm in both mouse and human models (S. J. Bedford-Guaus et al., 2011; Sanusi et al., 2015). Furthermore, injection of recombinant PLCζ yielded higher blastocyst development rates compare to Ca^{2+} ionophore treatment (Sanusi et al., 2015), indicating that PLCζ therapeutic regimens would be more effective in treating OAD compared to current AOA protocols.

In addition to potential therapeutic applications, numerous studies have now attempted to establish diagnostic applications of sperm PLCζ in humans, largely employing an immunocytological approach, associating defective/abnormal expression and localization patterns of PLCζ in multiple male-specific conditions (Azad, Nazarian, Ghaffari Novin, Masteri Farahani, Piryaei, & Heidari, 2018; Azad, Nazarian, Ghaffari Novin, Masteri Farahani, Piryaei, Heidari, et al., 2018; Escoffier et al., 2016; Escoffier et al., 2015; Janghorban-Laricheh et al., 2016; J. Kashir et al., 2010; Nikiforaki et al., 2014; Park et al., 2015; Marziyeh Tavalaee, Kiani-Esfahani, et al., 2017; Tavalaee et al., 2017; Tavalaee et al., 2018; Tavalaee, Parivar, Shahverdi, Ghaedi, & Nasr-Esfahani, 2017). However, despite such growing numbers of studies, consistent motifs between PLCζ and general sperm parameters and fertility outcomes have yet to be identified. Perhaps a causative factor underlying this is that the majority of antibodies employed to study PLCζ in humans have exhibited non-specificity and inconsistency between various studies (Escoffier et al., 2016; Escoffier et al., 2015; Heytens et al., 2009; Yoon et al., 2008), making it difficult to distinguish between PLCζ and other proteins upon immunocytological analysis.

Furthermore, (Kashir et al., 2016) indicated that specific antigen unmasking/retrieval protocols improved the visualization efficacy of PLCζ in mammalian sperm, suggesting that previous studies examining PLCζ localization may require re-examination, particularly in studies employing an immunofluorescence approach to quantify levels of PLCζ. Conversely, however, application of AUM was also found to differentially alter levels of observable PLCζ from individual human patients, raising questions as to whether application of AUM would potentially alter diagnostic outcomes.

CONCLUSION

PLCζ has rapidly gained wide acceptance as the 'soluble sperm factor', with numerous independent studies from around the world concluding that PLCζ is both necessary and sufficient to trigger Ca^{2+} oscillations at oocyte activation. Numerous clinical associations have now also been reported that directly link male infertility and OAD with reduced/absent expression levels and mutated forms of PLCζ, with further studies also implicating the involvement of PLCζ in determining the competency of subsequent embryogenesis. A number of clinical reports now collectively suggest that a very wide range of male conditions of infertility may be underscored by deficiencies and abnormalities in sperm PLCζ, or at the very least may be accompanied by such abrogation. It is thus clear that potentially numerous cases of male infertility may stand to benefit from the application of PLCζ as a therapeutic and diagnostic. However, while PLCζ exhibits great clinical promise for potentially a wide range of male infertility prognoses, research and clinical applications have been limited, preventing a methodical analysis of such potential. Such issues would require urgent addressing with specific tools before such examinations can be applied clinically.

REFERENCES

Aarabi, M., Qin, Z., Xu, W., Mewburn, J. & Oko, R. (2009). Sperm-borne protein, PAWP, initiates zygotic development in Xenopus laevis by eliciting intracellular calcium release. *Molecular Reproduction and Development*, n/a-n/a. doi:10.1002/mrd.21140.

Aarabi, M., Yu, Y., Xu, W., Tse, M. Y., Pang, S. C., Yi, Y. J. & Oko, R. (2012). The testicular and epididymal expression profile of PLCζ in mouse and human does not support its role as a sperm-borne oocyte activating factor. *PloS one*, *7*(3), e33496-e33496. doi:10.1371/journal.pone.0033496.

Agarwal, A., Panner Selvam, M. K. & Baskaran, S. (2020). Proteomic Analyses of Human Sperm Cells: Understanding the Role of Proteins and Molecular Pathways Affecting Male Reproductive Health. *International journal of molecular sciences*, *21*(5), 1621. doi:10.3390/ijms21051621.

Agarwal, A., Sharma, R., Durairajanayagam, D., Ayaz, A., Cui, Z., Willard, B. & Sabanegh, E. (2015). Major protein alterations in spermatozoa from infertile men with unilateral varicocele. *Reproductive biology and endocrinology : RB&E*, *13*, 8-8. doi:10.1186/s12958-015-0007-2.

Agarwal, A., Sharma, R., Durairajanayagam, D., Cui, Z., Ayaz, A., Gupta, S. & Sabanegh, E. (2015). Differential Proteomic Profiling of Spermatozoal Proteins of Infertile Men With Unilateral or Bilateral Varicocele. *Urology*, *85*(3), 580-588. doi:10.1016/j.urology.2014.11.030.

Aghajanpour, S., Ghaedi, K., Salamian, A., Deemeh, M. R., Tavalaee, M., Moshtaghian, J. & Nasr-Esfahani, M. H. (2011). Quantitative expression of phospholipase C zeta, as an index to assess fertilization potential of a semen sample. *Human Reproduction*, *26*(11), 2950-2956. doi:10.1093/humrep/der285.

Ahmadi, A. & Ng, S. C. (1999). Fertilizing ability of DNA-damaged spermatozoa. *The Journal of Experimental Zoology*, *284*(6), 696-704. doi:10.1002/(sici)1097-010x(19991101)284:6<696::aid-jez11>3.0.co;2-e.

Alvarez Sedo, C., Rawe, V. Y. & Chemes, H. E. (2012). Acrosomal biogenesis in human globozoospermia: immunocytochemical, ultrastructural and proteomic studies. *Human Reproduction*, *27*(7), 1912-1921. doi:10.1093/humrep/des126.

Alvarez Sedó, C., Bilinski, M., Lorenzi, D., Uriondo, H., Noblía, F., Longobucco, V. & Nodar, F. (2017). Effect of sperm DNA fragmentation on embryo development: clinical and biological aspects. *JBRA assisted reproduction*, *21*(4), 343-350. doi:10.5935/1518-0557.20170061.

Amdani, S. N., Yeste, M., Jones, C. & Coward, K. (2016). Phospholipase C zeta (PLCζ) and male infertility: Clinical update and topical developments. *Advances in Biological Regulation*, *61*, 58-67. doi:10.1016/j.jbior.2015.11.009.

Azad, N., Nazarian, H., Ghaffari Novin, M., Masteri Farahani, R., Piryaei, A. & Heidari, M. H. (2018). Phospholipase C zeta parameters in sperm from polymorphic teratozoospermic men. *Annals of Anatomy - Anatomischer Anzeiger*, *215*, 63-70. doi:10.1016/j.aanat.2017.09.007.

Azad, N., Nazarian, H., Ghaffari Novin, M., Masteri Farahani, R., Piryaei, A., Heidari, M. H. & Abdollahpour Alitappeh, M. (2018). Oligoasthenoteratozoospermic (OAT) men display altered phospholipase C ζ (PLCζ) localization and a lower percentage of sperm cells expressing PLCζ and post-acrosomal sheath WW domain-binding protein (PAWP). *Bosnian journal of basic medical sciences*, *18*(2), 178-184. doi:10.17305/bjbms.2017.2208.

Babayev, S., Park, C. & Bukulmez, O. (2014). Intracytoplasmic Sperm Injection Indications: How Rigorous? *Seminars in Reproductive Medicine*, *32*(04), 283-290. doi:10.1055/s-0034-1375180.

Barak, Y., Kogosowski, A., Goldman, S., Soffer, Y., Gonen, Y. & Tesarik, J. (1998). Pregnancy and birth after transfer of embryos that developed from single-nucleated zygotes obtained by injection of round spermatids into oocytes. *Fertility and Sterility*, *70*(1), 67-70. doi:10.1016/s0015-0282(98)00106-x.

Barratt, C. L. R., Aitken, R. J., Bjorndahl, L., Carrell, D. T., de Boer, P., Kvist, U. & Zini, A. (2010). Sperm DNA: organization, protection and vulnerability: from basic science to clinical applications--a position report. *Human Reproduction*, *25*(4), 824-838. doi:10.1093/humrep/dep465.

Bedford-Guaus, S. J., McPartlin, L. A., Xie, J., Westmiller, S. L., Buffone, M. G. & Roberson, M. S. (2011). Molecular Cloning and Characterization of Phospholipase C Zeta in Equine Sperm and Testis Reveals Species-Specific Differences in Expression of Catalytically Active Protein1. *Biology of Reproduction*, *85*(1), 78-88. doi:10.1095/biolreprod.110.089466.

Bedford-Guaus, S. J., Yoon, S. Y., Fissore, R. A., Choi, Y. H. & Hinrichs, K. (2008). Microinjection of mouse phospholipase Cζ complementary RNA into mare oocytes induces long-lasting intracellular calcium oscillations and embryonic development. *Reproduction, Fertility and Development*, *20*(8), 875. doi:10.1071/rd08115.

Bi, Y., Xu, W. M., Wong, H. Y., Zhu, H., Zhou, Z. M., Chan, H. C. & Sha, J. H. (2009). NYD-SP27, a novel intrinsic decapacitation factor in sperm. *Asian journal of andrology*, *11*(2), 229-239. doi:10.1038/aja.2009.6.

Bieniek, J. M., Drabovich, A. P. & Lo, K. C. (2016). Seminal biomarkers for the evaluation of male infertility. *Asian journal of andrology*, *18*(3), 426-433. doi:10.4103/1008-682X.175781.

Botezatu, A., Socolov, R., Socolov, D., Iancu, I. V. & Anton, G. (2014). Methylation pattern of methylene tetrahydrofolate reductase and small nuclear ribonucleoprotein polypeptide N promoters in oligoasthenospermia: a case-control study. *Reproductive BioMedicine Online*, *28*(2), 225-231. doi:10.1016/j.rbmo. 2013.10.010.

Boulet, S. L., Mehta, A., Kissin, D. M., Warner, L., Kawwass, J. F. & Jamieson, D. J. (2015). Trends in use of and reproductive outcomes associated with intracytoplasmic sperm injection. *JAMA*, *313*(3), 255-263. doi:10.1001/jama.2014.17985.

Brind, S., Swann, K. & Carroll, J. (2000). Inositol 1,4,5-Trisphosphate Receptors Are Downregulated in Mouse Oocytes in Response to Sperm or Adenophostin A but Not to Increases in Intracellular Ca2+ or Egg Activation. *Developmental Biology*, *223*(2), 251-265. doi:10.1006/dbio.2000.9728.

Cao, X., Cui, Y., Zhang, X., Lou, J., Zhou, J., Bei, H. & Wei, R. (2018). Proteomic profile of human spermatozoa in healthy and asthenozoospermic individuals. *Reproductive biology and endocrinology: RB&E*, *16*(1), 16-16. doi:10.1186/s12958-018-0334-1.

Chambers, G. M., Wand, H., Macaldowie, A., Chapman, M. G., Farquhar, C. M., Bowman, M. & Ledger, W. (2016). Population trends and live birth rates associated with common ART treatment strategies. *Human Reproduction*, *31*(11), 2632-2641. doi:10.1093/humrep/dew232.

Chan, C. C., Sun, G. H., Shui, H. A. & Wu, G. J. (2013). Differential Spermatozoal Protein Expression Profiles in Men With Varicocele Compared to Control Subjects: Upregulation of Heat Shock Proteins 70 and 90 in Varicocele. *Urology*, *81*(6), 1379.e1371-1379.e1378. doi:10.1016/j.urology.2013.01.031.

Chansel-Debordeaux, L., Dandieu, S., Bechoua, S. & Jimenez, C. (2015). Reproductive outcome in globozoospermic men: update and prospects. *Andrology*, *3*(6), 1022-1034. doi:10.1111/andr.12081.

Collins, J. K. & Jones, K. T. (2016). DNA damage responses in mammalian oocytes. *Reproduction*, *152*(1), R15-R22. doi:10.1530/rep-16-0069.

Cousens, S., Blencowe, H., Stanton, C., Chou, D., Ahmed, S., Steinhardt, L. & Lawn, J. E. (2011). National, regional, and worldwide estimates of stillbirth rates in 2009 with trends since 1995: a systematic analysis. *The Lancet*, *377*(9774), 1319-1330. doi:10.1016/s0140-6736(10)62310-0.

Coward, K., Campos-Mendoza, A., Larman, M., Hibbitt, O., McAndrew, B., Bromage, N. & Parrington, J. (2003). Teleost fish spermatozoa contain a cytosolic protein factor that induces calcium release in sea urchin egg homogenates and triggers calcium oscillations when injected into mouse oocytes. *Biochemical and Biophysical Research Communications*, *305*(2), 299-304. doi:10.1016/s0006-291x(03)00753-8.

Coward, K., Owen, H., Tunwell, R., Swann, K. & Parrington, J. (2007). Phospholipid binding properties and functional characterization of a sea urchin phospholipase Cδ in urchin and mouse eggs. *Biochemical and Biophysical Research Communications*, *357*(4), 964-970. doi:10.1016/j.bbrc.2007.04.050.

Coward, K., Ponting, C. P., Chang, H. Y., Hibbitt, O., Savolainen, P., Jones, K. T. & Parrington, J. (2005). Phospholipase Cζ, the trigger of egg activation in mammals, is present in a non-mammalian species. *Reproduction*, *130*(2), 157-163. doi:10.1530/rep.1.00707.

Coward, K., Ponting, C. P., Zhang, N., Young, C., Huang, C. J., Chou, C. M. & Parrington, J. (2011). Identification and functional analysis of an ovarian form of the egg activation factor phospholipase C zeta (PLCζ) in pufferfish. *Molecular Reproduction and Development*, *78*(1), 48-56. doi:10.1002/mrd.21262.

Cox, L. J., Larman, M. G., Saunders, C. M., Hashimoto, K., Swann, K. & Lai, F. A. (2002). Sperm phospholipase Czeta from humans and cynomolgus monkeys triggers Ca2+ oscillations, activation and development of mouse oocytes. *Reproduction*, 611-623. doi:10.1530/rep.0.1240611.

Cruz, M., Gadea, B., Garrido, N., Pedersen, K. S., Martínez, M., Pérez-Cano, I. & Meseguer, M. (2011). Embryo quality, blastocyst and ongoing pregnancy rates in oocyte donation patients whose embryos were monitored by time-lapse imaging. *Journal of assisted reproduction and genetics*, *28*(7), 569-573. doi:10.1007/s10815-011-9549-1.

Dai, J., Dai, C., Guo, J., Zheng, W., Zhang, T., Li, Y. & Lin, G. (2019). Novel homozygous variations in PLCZ1 lead to poor or failed fertilization characterized by abnormal localization patterns of PLCζ in sperm. *Clinical Genetics*, *97*(2), 347-351. doi:10.1111/cge.13636.

Dam, A. H. D. M., Feenstra, I., Westphal, J. R., Ramos, L., van Golde, R. J. T. & Kremer, J. A. M. (2006). Globozoospermia revisited. *Human Reproduction Update*, *13*(1), 63-75. doi:10.1093/humupd/dml047.

De Braekeleer, M., Nguyen, M. H., Morel, F. & Perrin, A. (2015). Genetic aspects of monomorphic teratozoospermia: a review. *Journal of assisted reproduction and genetics*, *32*(4), 615-623. doi:10.1007/s10815-015-0433-2.

De Vos, A., Van De Velde, H., Joris, H., Verheyen, G., Devroey, P. & Van Steirteghem, A. (2003). Influence of individual sperm morphology on fertilization, embryo morphology, and pregnancy outcome of intracytoplasmic sperm injection. *Fertility and Sterility*, *79*(1), 42-48. doi:10.1016/s0015-0282(02)04571-5.

Desai, N., Ploskonka, S., Goodman, L. R., Austin, C., Goldberg, J. & Falcone, T. (2014). Analysis of embryo morphokinetics, multinucleation and cleavage anomalies using continuous time-lapse monitoring in blastocyst transfer cycles. *Reproductive biology and endocrinology: RB&E*, *12*, 54-54. doi:10.1186/1477-7827-12-54.

Deyhoul, N., Mohamaddoost, T. & Hosseini, M. (2017). Infertility-Related Risk Factors: A Systematic Review. *International Journal of Women's Health and Reproduction Sciences*, *5*(1), 24-29. doi:10.15296/ijwhr.2017.05.

Dong, J. B., Tang, T. S. & Sun, F. Z. (2000). Xenopus and Chicken Sperm Contain a Cytosolic Soluble Protein Factor Which Can Trigger Calcium Oscillations in Mouse Eggs. *Biochemical and Biophysical Research Communications*, *268*(3), 947-951. doi:10.1006/bbrc.2000.2218.

Drabovich, A. P., Dimitromanolakis, A., Saraon, P., Soosaipillai, A., Batruch, I., Mullen, B. & Diamandis, E. P. (2013). Differential Diagnosis of Azoospermia with Proteomic Biomarkers ECM1 and TEX101 Quantified in Seminal Plasma. *Science Translational Medicine*, *5*(212), 212ra160-212ra160. doi:10.1126/scitrans lmed.3006260.

Ducibella, T. & Fissore, R. (2008). The roles of Ca2+, downstream protein kinases, and oscillatory signaling in regulating fertilization and the activation of development. *Developmental biology*, *315*(2), 257-279. doi:10.1016/j.ydbio.2007.12.012.

Ducibella, T., Huneau, D., Angelichio, E., Xu, Z., Schultz, R. M., Kopf, G. S. & Ozil, J. P. (2002). Egg-to-Embryo Transition Is Driven by Differential Responses to Ca2+ Oscillation Number. *Developmental Biology*, *250*(2), 280-291. doi:10.1006/dbio.2002.0788.

Ducibella, T., Schultz, R. & Ozil, J. (2006). Role of calcium signals in early development. *Seminars in Cell & Developmental Biology*, *17*(2), 324-332. doi:10.1016/j.semcdb.2006.02.010.

Dyer, S. J. (2007). The value of children in African countries – insights from studies on infertility. *Journal of Psychosomatic Obstetrics & Gynecology*, *28*(2), 69-77. doi:10.1080/01674820701409959.

Escoffier, J., Lee, H. C., Yassine, S., Zouari, R., Martinez, G., Karaouzène, T. & Arnoult, C. (2016). Homozygous mutation of PLCZ1 leads to defective human oocyte activation and infertility that is not rescued by the WW-binding protein PAWP. *Human molecular genetics*, *25*(5), 878-891. doi:10.1093/hmg/ddv617.

Escoffier, J., Yassine, S., Lee, H. C., Martinez, G., Delaroche, J., Coutton, C. & Arnoult, C. (2015). Subcellular localization of phospholipase Cζ in human sperm and its absence in DPY19L2-deficient sperm are consistent with its role in oocyte activation. *Molecular human reproduction*, *21*(2), 157-168. doi:10.1093/molehr/gau098.

Esteves, S. C. (2015). Clinical management of infertile men with nonobstructive azoospermia. *Asian journal of andrology*, *17*(3), 459-470. doi:10.4103/1008-682X.148719.

Esteves, S. C., Roque, M., Bedoschi, G., Haahr, T. & Humaidan, P. (2018). Intracytoplasmic sperm injection for male infertility and consequences for offspring. *Nature Reviews Urology*, *15*(9), 535-562. doi:10.1038/s41585-018-0051-8.

Fauque, P., Léandri, R., Merlet, F., Juillard, J. C., Epelboin, S., Guibert, J. & Patrat, C. (2007). Pregnancy outcome and live birth after IVF and ICSI according to embryo quality. *Journal of assisted reproduction and genetics*, *24*(5), 159-165. doi:10.1007/s10815-007-9115-z.

Fawzy, M., Emad, M., Mahran, A., Sabry, M., Fetih, A. N., Abdelghafar, H. & Rasheed, S. (2018). Artificial oocyte activation with SrCl2 or calcimycin after ICSI improves clinical and embryological outcomes compared with ICSI alone: results of a randomized clinical trial. *Human Reproduction*, *33*(9), 1636-1644. doi:10.1093/humrep/dey258.

Ferrer-Vaquer, A., Barragan, M., Freour, T., Vernaeve, V. & Vassena, R. (2016). PLCζ sequence, protein levels, and distribution in human sperm do not correlate with semen characteristics and fertilization rates after ICSI. *Journal of assisted reproduction and genetics*, *33*(6), 747-756. doi:10.1007/s10815-016-0718-0.

Fujimoto, S., Yoshida, N., Fukui, T., Amanai, M., Isobe, T., Itagaki, C. & Perry, A. C. F. (2004). Mammalian phospholipase Cζ induces oocyte activation from the sperm perinuclear matrix. *Developmental Biology*, *274*(2), 370-383. doi:10.1016/j.ydbio.2004.07.025.

Fulton, B. P. & Whittingham, D. G. (1978). Activation of mammalian oocytes by intracellular injection of calcium. *Nature*, *273*(5658), 149-151. doi:10.1038/273149a0.

Gawecka, J. E., Marh, J., Ortega, M., Yamauchi, Y., Ward, M. A. & Ward, W. S. (2013). Mouse zygotes respond to severe sperm DNA damage by delaying paternal DNA replication and embryonic development. *PloS one*, *8*(2), e56385-e56385. doi:10.1371/journal.pone.0056385.

Gawecka, J. E., Ribas-Maynou, J., Benet, J. & Ward, W. S. (2015). A model for the control of DNA integrity by the sperm nuclear matrix. *Asian journal of andrology*, *17*(4), 610-615. doi:10.4103/1008-682X.153853

Genescà, A., Caballín, M. R., Miró, R., Benet, J., Germà, J. R. & Egozcue, J. (1992). Repair of human sperm chromosome aberrations in the hamster egg. *Human Genetics*, *89*(2). doi:10.1007/bf00217120.

Gianaroli, L., Selman, H. A., Magli, M. C., Colpi, G., Fortini, D. & Ferraretti, A. P. (1999). Birth of a healthy infant after conception with round spermatids isolated from cryopreserved testicular tissue. *Fertility and Sterility*, *72*(3), 539-541. doi:10.1016/s0015-0282(99)00285-x.

González-Marín, C., Gosálvez, J. & Roy, R. (2012). Types, causes, detection and repair of DNA fragmentation in animal and human sperm cells. *International journal of molecular sciences*, *13*(11), 14026-14052. doi:10.3390/ijms131114026.

Grasa, P., Coward, K., Young, C. & Parrington, J. (2008). The pattern of localization of the putative oocyte activation factor, phospholipase C, in uncapacitated, capacitated, and ionophore-treated human spermatozoa. *Human Reproduction*, *23*(11), 2513-2522. doi:10.1093/humrep/den280.

Gurunath, S., Pandian, Z., Anderson, R. A. & Bhattacharya, S. (2011). Defining infertility—a systematic review of prevalence studies. *Human Reproduction Update*, *17*(5), 575-588. doi:10.1093/humupd/dmr015.

Hachem, A., Godwin, J., Ruas, M., Lee, H. C., Ferrer Buitrago, M., Ardestani, G. & Parrington, J. (2017). PLCζ is the physiological trigger of the Ca(2+) oscillations that induce embryogenesis in mammals but conception can occur in its absence. *Development (Cambridge, England), 144*(16), 2914-2924. doi:10.1242/dev.150227.

Hashemitabar, M., Sabbagh, S., Orazizadeh, M., Ghadiri, A. & Bahmanzadeh, M. (2015). A proteomic analysis on human sperm tail: comparison between normozoospermia and asthenozoospermia. *Journal of assisted reproduction and genetics, 32*(6), 853-863. doi:10.1007/s10815-015-0465-7.

Herwig, R., Knoll, C., Planyavsky, M., Pourbiabany, A., Greilberger, J. & Bennett, K. L. (2013). Proteomic analysis of seminal plasma from infertile patients with oligoasthenoteratozoospermia due to oxidative stress and comparison with fertile volunteers. *Fertility and Sterility, 100*(2), 355-366.e352. doi:10.1016/j.fertnstert.2013.03.048.

Heytens, E., Parrington, J., Coward, K., Young, C., Lambrecht, S., Yoon, S. Y. & De Sutter, P. (2009). Reduced amounts and abnormal forms of phospholipase C zeta (PLC) in spermatozoa from infertile men. *Human Reproduction, 24*(10), 2417-2428. doi:10.1093/humrep/dep207.

Hirabayashi, M., Kato, M. & Hochi, S. (2008). Factors Affecting Full-Term Development of Rat Oocytes Microinjected with Fresh or Cryopreserved Round Spermatids. *Experimental Animals, 57*(4), 401-405. doi:10.1538/expanim.57.401.

Hirabayashi, M., Kato, M., Kitada, K., Ohnami, N., Hirao, M. & Hochi, S. (2009). Activation regimens for full-term development of rabbit oocytes injected with round spermatids. *Molecular Reproduction and Development, 76*(6), 573-579. doi:10.1002/mrd.20984.

Horner, V. L. & Wolfner, M. F. (2008). Transitioning from egg to embryo: Triggers and mechanisms of egg activation. *Developmental Dynamics, 237*(3), 527-544. doi:10.1002/dvdy.21454.

Hosseinifar, H., Gourabi, H., Salekdeh, G. H., Alikhani, M., Mirshahvaladi, S., Sabbaghian, M. & Gilani, M. A. S. (2013). Study of Sperm Protein Profile in Men With and Without Varicocele Using

Two-Dimensional Gel Electrophoresis. *Urology*, *81*(2), 293-300. doi:10.1016/j.urology.2012.06.027.

Igarashi, H., Knott, J. G., Schultz, R. M. & Williams, C. J. (2007). Alterations of PLCbeta1 in mouse eggs change calcium oscillatory behavior following fertilization. *Developmental biology*, *312*(1), 321-330. doi:10.1016/j.ydbio.2007.09.028.

Irvine, D. S. (1998). Epidemiology and aetiology of male infertility. *Human Reproduction*, *13*(suppl 1), 33-44. doi:10.1093/humrep/13.suppl_1.33.

Ito, J., Parrington, J. & Fissore, R. A. (2011). PLCζ and its role as a trigger of development in vertebrates. *Molecular Reproduction and Development*, *78*(10-11), 846-853. doi:10.1002/mrd.21359.

Ito, M., Shikano, T., Oda, S., Horiguchi, T., Tanimoto, S., Awaji, T. & Miyazaki, S. (2008). Difference in Ca2+ Oscillation-Inducing Activity and Nuclear Translocation Ability of PLCZ1, an Egg-Activating Sperm Factor Candidate, Between Mouse, Rat, Human, and Medaka Fish1. *Biology of Reproduction*, *78*(6), 1081-1090. doi:10.1095/biolreprod.108.067801.

Janghorban-Laricheh, E., Ghazavi-Khorasgani, N., Tavalaee, M., Zohrabi, D., Abbasi, H. & Nasr-Esfahani, M. H. (2016). An association between sperm PLCζ levels and varicocele? *Journal of assisted reproduction and genetics*, *33*(12), 1649-1655. doi:10.1007/s10815-016-0802-5.

Javed, M., Esfandiari, N. & Casper, R. F. (2011). Retraction notice to "Failed fertilization after clinical intracytoplasmic sperm injection" [RBMO 20 (2010) 56–67]. *Reproductive BioMedicine Online*, *23*(6), 806. doi:10.1016/j.rbmo.2011.09.001.

Jellerette, T., He, C. L., Wu, H., Parys, J. B. & Fissore, R. A. (2000). Down-regulation of the Inositol 1,4,5-Trisphosphate Receptor in Mouse Eggs Following Fertilization or Parthenogenetic Activation. *Developmental Biology*, *223*(2), 238-250. doi:10.1006/dbio.2000.9675.

Jones, K. T., Carroll, J. & Whittingham, D. G. (1995). Ionomycin, Thapsigargin, Ryanodine, and Sperm Induced Ca2+Release Increase during Meiotic Maturation of Mouse Oocytes. *Journal of Biological Chemistry*, *270*(12), 6671-6677. doi:10.1074/jbc.270.12.6671.

Jones, K. T., Soeller, C. & Cannell, M. B. (1998). The passage of Ca2+ and fluorescent markers between the sperm and egg after fusion in the mouse. *Development*, *125*(23), 4627-4635.

Kaewmala, K., Uddin, M. J., Cinar, M. U., Große-Brinkhaus, C., Jonas, E., Tesfaye, D. & Schellander, K. (2011). Investigation into Association and Expression of PLCz and COX-2 as Candidate Genes for Boar Sperm Quality and Fertility. *Reproduction in Domestic Animals*, *47*(2), 213-223. doi:10.1111/j.1439-0531.2011.01831.x.

Kamali-Dolat Abadi, M., Tavalaee, M., Shahverdi, A. & Nasr-Esfahani, M. H. (2016). Evaluation of PLCζ and PAWP Expression in Globozoospermic Individuals. *Cell J*, *18*(3), 438-445. doi:10.22074/cellj.2016.4572.

Kashir, J. (2020). Increasing associations between defects in phospholipase C zeta and conditions of male infertility: not just ICSI failure? *Journal of Assisted Reproduction and Genetics*. doi:10.1007/s10815-020-01748-z.

Kashir, J., Buntwal, L., Nomikos, M., Calver, B. L., Stamatiadis, P., Ashley, P. & Lai, F. A. (2016). Antigen unmasking enhances visualization efficacy of the oocyte activation factor, phospholipase C zeta, in mammalian sperm. *Molecular Human Reproduction*, *23*(1), 54-67. doi:10.1093/molehr/gaw073.

Kashir, J., Heindryckx, B., Jones, C., De Sutter, P., Parrington, J. & Coward, K. (2010). Oocyte activation, phospholipase C zeta and human infertility. *Human Reproduction Update*, *16*(6), 690-703. doi:10.1093/humupd/dmq018.

Kashir, J., Heynen, A., Jones, C., Durrans, C., Craig, J., Gadea, J. & Coward, K. (2011). Effects of cryopreservation and density-gradient washing on phospholipase C zeta concentrations in human spermatozoa. *Reproductive BioMedicine Online*, *23*(2), 263-267. doi:10.1016/j.rbmo.2011.04.006.

Kashir, J., Jones, C., Lee, H. C., Rietdorf, K., Nikiforaki, D., Durrans, C. & Coward, K. (2011). Loss of activity mutations in phospholipase C zeta (PLCζ) abolishes calcium oscillatory ability of human recombinant protein in mouse oocytes. *Human reproduction (Oxford, England)*, *26*(12), 3372-3387. doi:10.1093/humrep/der336.

Kashir, J., Jones, C., Mounce, G., Ramadan, W. M., Lemmon, B., Heindryckx, B. & Coward, K. (2013). Variance in total levels of phospholipase C zeta (PLC-ζ) in human sperm may limit the applicability of quantitative immunofluorescent analysis as a diagnostic indicator of oocyte activation capability. *Fertility and Sterility*, *99*(1), 107-117.e103. doi:10.1016/j.fertnstert.2012.09.001.

Kashir, J., Konstantinidis, M., Jones, C., Heindryckx, B., De Sutter, P., Parrington, J. & Coward, K. (2012). Characterization of two heterozygous mutations of the oocyte activation factor phospholipase C zeta (PLCζ) from an infertile man by use of minisequencing of individual sperm and expression in somatic cells. *Fertility and Sterility*, *98*(2), 423-431. doi:10.1016/j.fertnstert.2012.05.002.

Kashir, J., Konstantinidis, M., Jones, C., Lemmon, B., Lee, H. C., Hamer, R. & Coward, K. (2012). A maternally inherited autosomal point mutation in human phospholipase C zeta (PLCζ) leads to male infertility. *Human reproduction (Oxford, England)*, *27*(1), 222-231. doi:10.1093/humrep/der384.

Kashir, J., Mistry, B. V., BuSaleh, L., Abu-Dawas, R., Nomikos, M., Ajlan, A. & Coskun, S. (2020). Phospholipase C zeta profiles are indicative of optimal sperm parameters and fertilization success in patients undergoing fertility treatment. *Andrology*. doi:10.1111/andr.12796.

Kashir, J., Nomikos, M., Lai, F. A. & Swann, K. (2014). Sperm-induced Ca2+ release during egg activation in mammals. *Biochemical and Biophysical Research Communications*, *450*(3), 1204-1211. doi:10.1016/j.bbrc.2014.04.078.

Kashir, J., Sermondade, N., Sifer, C., Oo, S. L., Jones, C., Mounce, G. & Coward, K. (2012). Motile sperm organelle morphology evaluation-selected globozoospermic human sperm with an acrosomal bud exhibits novel patterns and higher levels of phospholipase C zeta. *Human Reproduction*, *27*(11), 3150-3160. doi:10.1093/humrep/des312.

Kimura, Y. & Yanagimachi, R. (1995). Mouse oocytes injected with testicular spermatozoa or round spermatids can develop into normal offspring. *Development*, *121*(8), 2397-2405.

Kline, D. & Kline, J. T. (1992). Repetitive calcium transients and the role of calcium in exocytosis and cell cycle activation in the mouse egg. *Developmental Biology*, *149*(1), 80-89. doi:10.1016/0012-1606(92)90265-i.

Kline, J. T. & Kline, D. (1994). Regulation of Intracellular Calcium in the Mouse Egg: Evidence for Inositol Trisphosphate-Induced Calcium Release, but not Calcium-Induced Calcium Release1. *Biology of Reproduction*, *50*(1), 193-203. doi:10.1095/biolreprod50.1.193.

Knez, K., Zorn, B., Tomazevic, T., Vrtacnik-Bokal, E. & Virant-Klun, I. (2011). The IMSI procedure improves poor embryo development in the same infertile couples with poor semen quality: a comparative prospective randomized study. *Reproductive biology and endocrinology: RB&E*, *9*, 123-123. doi:10.1186/1477-7827-9-123.

Knott, J. G., Kurokawa, M., Fissore, R. A., Schultz, R. M. & Williams, C. J. (2005). Transgenic RNA Interference Reveals Role for Mouse Sperm Phospholipase Cζ in Triggering Ca2+ Oscillations During Fertilization1. *Biology of Reproduction*, *72*(4), 992-996. doi:10.1095/biolreprod.104.036244.

Kouchi, Z., Shikano, T., Nakamura, Y., Shirakawa, H., Fukami, K. & Miyazaki, S. (2005). The Role of EF-hand Domains and C2 Domain in Regulation of Enzymatic Activity of Phospholipase Cζ. *Journal of Biological Chemistry*, *280*(22), 21015-21021. doi:10.1074/jbc.m412123200.

Kumar, N. & Singh, A. K. (2015). Trends of male factor infertility, an important cause of infertility: A review of literature. *Journal of human reproductive sciences*, *8*(4), 191-196. doi:10.4103/0974-1208.170370.

Kurokawa, M., Sato, K. i., Wu, H., He, C., Malcuit, C., Black, S. J. & Fissore, R. A. (2005). Functional, biochemical, and chromatographic characterization of the complete [Ca2+]i oscillation-inducing activity of porcine sperm. *Developmental Biology*, *285*(2), 376-392. doi:10.1016/j.ydbio.2005.06.029.

Kyozuka, K., Deguchi, R., Mohri, T. & Miyazaki, S. (1998). Injection of sperm extract mimics spatiotemporal dynamics of Ca2+ responses and progression of meiosis at fertilization of ascidian oocytes. *Development*, *125*(20), 4099-4105.

Lewis, S. E. M. & Aitken, R. J. (2005). DNA damage to spermatozoa has impacts on fertilization and pregnancy. *Cell and Tissue Research*, *322*(1), 33-41. doi:10.1007/s00441-005-1097-5.

Liao, T. T., Xiang, Z., Zhu, W. B. & Fan, L. Q. (2009). Proteome analysis of round-headed and normal spermatozoa by 2-D fluorescence difference gel electrophoresis and mass spectrometry. *Asian journal of andrology*, *11*(6), 683-693. doi:10.1038/aja.2009.59.

Liu, J., Nagy, Z., Joris, H., Tournaye, H., Devroey, P. & Van Steirteghem, A. (1995). Andrology: Successful fertilization and establishment of pregnancies after intracytoplasmic sperm injection in patients with globozoospermia. *Human Reproduction*, *10*(3), 626-629. doi:10.1093/oxfordjournals.humrep.a136000.

Liu, X., Wang, W., Zhu, P., Wang, J., Wang, Y., Wang, X. & Liu, F. (2018). In-depth quantitative proteome analysis of seminal plasma from men with oligoasthenozoospermia and normozoospermia. *Reproductive BioMedicine Online*, *37*(4), 467-479. doi:10.1016/j.rbmo.2018.06.025.

Loren, J. & Lacham-Kaplan, O. (2006). The employment of strontium to activate mouse oocytes: effects on spermatid-injection outcome. *Reproduction*, *131*(2), 259-267. doi:10.1530/rep.1.00894.

Loutradi, K. E., Tarlatzis, B. C., Goulis, D. G., Zepiridis, L., Pagou, T., Chatziioannou, E. & Bontis, I. (2006). The effects of sperm quality on embryo development after intracytoplasmic sperm injection. *Journal of assisted reproduction and genetics*, *23*(2), 69-74. doi:10.1007/s10815-006-9022-8.

Ludwig, M., Strik, D., Al-Hasani, S. & Diedrich, K. (1999). No transfer in a planned ICSI cycle: we cannot overcome some basic rules of human reproduction. *European Journal of Obstetrics & Gynecology and Reproductive Biology*, *87*(1), 3-11. doi:10.1016/s0301-2115(99)00071-8.

Lundin, K., Sjögren, A., Nilsson, L. & Hamberger, L. (1994). Fertilization and pregnancy after intracytoplasmic microinjection of acrosomeless spermatozoa**Supported by the Swedish Medical Research Council, grants no. 2873 and 05978, and by the Helge Ax:son Johnson Foundation, Stockholm, Sweden. *Fertility and Sterility*, *62*(6), 1266-1267. doi:10.1016/s0015-0282(16)57197-0.

Mahutte, N. G. & Arici, A. (2003). Failed fertilization: is it predictable? *Current Opinion in Obstetrics and Gynecology*, *15*(3), 211-218. doi:10.1097/00001703-200306000-00001.

Malcuit, C., Kurokawa, M. & Fissore, R. A. (2005). Calcium oscillations and mammalian egg activation. *Journal of Cellular Physiology*, *206*(3), 565-573. doi:10.1002/jcp.20471.

Manandhar, G. & Toshimori, K. (2003). Fate of Postacrosomal Perinuclear Theca Recognized by Monoclonal Antibody MN13 after Sperm Head Microinjection and Its Role in Oocyte Activation in Mice1. *Biology of Reproduction*, *68*(2), 655-663. doi:10.1095/biolreprod.102.006098.

Martin, J. H., Bromfield, E. G., Aitken, R. J., Lord, T. & Nixon, B. (2018). Double Strand Break DNA Repair occurs via Non-Homologous End-Joining in Mouse MII Oocytes. *Scientific reports*, *8*(1), 9685-9685. doi:10.1038/s41598-018-27892-2.

Martinez-Heredia, J., de Mateo, S., Vidal-Taboada, J. M., Ballesca, J. L. & Oliva, R. (2008). Identification of proteomic differences in asthenozoospermic sperm samples. *Human Reproduction*, *23*(4), 783-791. doi:10.1093/humrep/den024.

Mascarenhas, M. N., Flaxman, S. R., Boerma, T., Vanderpoel, S. & Stevens, G. A. (2012). National, regional, and global trends in infertility prevalence since 1990: a systematic analysis of 277 health surveys. *PLoS medicine*, *9*(12), e1001356-e1001356. doi:10.1371/journal.pmed.1001356.

Mejía-Flores, I., Chiquete-Félix, N., Palma-Lara, I., Uribe-Carvajal, S. & de Lourdes Juárez-Mosqueda, M. (2017). During capacitation in bull spermatozoa, actin and PLC-ζ undergo dynamic interactions. *Zygote*, *25*(5), 558-566. doi:10.1017/s0967199417000260.

Milewski, R., Szpila, M. & Ajduk, A. (2018). Dynamics of cytoplasm and cleavage divisions correlates with preimplantation embryo development. *Reproduction*, *155*(1), 1-14. doi:10.1530/rep-17-0230.

Miyazaki, S. & Ito, M. (2006). Calcium Signals for Egg Activation in Mammals. *Journal of Pharmacological Sciences*, *100*(5), 545-552. doi:10.1254/jphs.cpj06003x.

Miyazaki, S., Shirakawa, H., Nakada, K. & Honda, Y. (1993). Essential Role of the Inositol 1,4,5-Trisphosphate Receptor/Ca2+ Release

Channel in Ca2+ Waves and Ca2+ Oscillations at Fertilization of Mammalian Eggs. *Developmental Biology*, *158*(1), 62-78. doi:10.1006/dbio.1993.1168.

Miyazaki, S., Yuzaki, M., Nakada, K., Shirakawa, H., Nakanishi, S., Nakade, S. & Mikoshiba, K. (1992). Block of Ca2+ wave and Ca2+ oscillation by antibody to the inositol 1,4,5-trisphosphate receptor in fertilized hamster eggs. *Science*, *257*(5067), 251-255. doi:10.1126/science.1321497.

Mizushima, S., Takagi, S., Ono, T., Atsumi, Y., Tsukada, A., Saito, N. & Shimada, K. (2009). Phospholipase Cζ mRNA expression and its potency during spermatogenesis for activation of quail oocyte as a sperm factor. *Molecular Reproduction and Development*, *76*(12), 1200-1207. doi:10.1002/mrd.21097.

Montag, M., Köster, M., van der Ven, K., Bohlen, U. & van der Ven, H. (2012). The benefit of artificial oocyte activation is dependent on the fertilization rate in a previous treatment cycle. *Reproductive BioMedicine Online*, *24*(5), 521-526. doi:10.1016/j.rbmo.2012.02.002.

Mu, J., Zhang, Z., Wu, L., Fu, J., Chen, B., Yan, Z. & Sang, Q. (2020). The identification of novel mutations in PLCZ1 responsible for human fertilization failure and a therapeutic intervention by artificial oocyte activation. *Molecular Human Reproduction*, *26*(2), 80-87. doi:10.1093/molehr/gaaa003.

Murugesu, S., Saso, S., Jones, B. P., Bracewell-Milnes, T., Athanasiou, T., Mania, A. & Ben-Nagi, J. (2017). Does the use of calcium ionophore during artificial oocyte activation demonstrate an effect on pregnancy rate? A meta-analysis. *Fertility and Sterility*, *108*(3), 468-482.e463. doi:10.1016/j.fertnstert.2017.06.029.

Nader, N., Kulkarni, R. P., Dib, M. & Machaca, K. (2013). How to make a good egg! *Cell Calcium*, *53*(1), 41-54. doi:10.1016/j.ceca.2012.11.015.

Nakai, M., Ito, J., Sato, K. i., Noguchi, J., Kaneko, H., Kashiwazaki, N. & Kikuchi, K. (2011). Pre-treatment of sperm reduces success of ICSI in the pig. *Reproduction*, *142*(2), 285-293. doi:10.1530/rep-11-0073.

Nakano, Y. (1997). Spatiotemporal dynamics of intracellular calcium in the mouse egg injected with a spermatozoon. *Molecular Human Reproduction*, *3*(12), 1087-1093. doi:10.1093/molehr/3.12.1087.

Nicopoullos, J., Vicens-Morton, A., Lewis, S. E. M., Lee, K., Larsen, P., Ramsay, J. & Minhas, S. (2019). Novel use of COMET parameters of sperm DNA damage may increase its utility to diagnose male infertility and predict live births following both IVF and ICSI. *Human Reproduction*, *34*(10), 1915-1923. doi:10.1093/humrep/dez151.

Nikiforaki, D., Vanden Meerschaut, F., De Gheselle, S., Qian, C., Van den Abbeel, E., De Vos, W. H. & Heindryckx, B. (2014). Sperm involved in recurrent partial hydatidiform moles cannot induce the normal pattern of calcium oscillations. *Fertility and Sterility*, *102*(2), 581-588.e581. doi:10.1016/j.fertnstert.2014.05.004.

Nomikos, M., Blayney, L. M., Larman, M. G., Campbell, K., Rossbach, A., Saunders, C. M. & Lai, F. A. (2005). Role of Phospholipase C-ζ Domains in Ca2+-dependent Phosphatidylinositol 4,5-Bisphosphate Hydrolysis and Cytoplasmic Ca2+Oscillations. *Journal of Biological Chemistry*, *280*(35), 31011-31018. doi:10.1074/jbc.m500629200.

Nomikos, M., Elgmati, K., Theodoridou, M., Calver, B. L., Nounesis, G., Swann, K. & Lai, F. A. (2011). Phospholipase Cζ binding to PtdIns(4,5)P2 requires the XY-linker region. *Journal of cell science*, *124*(Pt 15), 2582-2590. doi:10.1242/jcs.083485.

Nomikos, M., Elgmati, K., Theodoridou, M., Georgilis, A., Gonzalez-Garcia, J. R., Nounesis, G. & Lai, F. A. (2011). Novel regulation of PLCζ activity via its XY-linker. *The Biochemical journal*, *438*(3), 427-432. doi:10.1042/BJ20110953.

Nomikos, M., Kashir, J., Swann, K. & Lai, F. A. (2013). Sperm PLCζ: From structure to Ca2+oscillations, egg activation and therapeutic potential. *FEBS Letters*, *587*(22), 3609-3616. doi:10.1016/j.febslet.2013.10.008.

Nomikos, M., Mulgrew-Nesbitt, A., Pallavi, P., Mihalyne, G., Zaitseva, I., Swann, K. & McLaughlin, S. (2007). Binding of Phosphoinositide-specific Phospholipase C-ζ (PLC-ζ) to Phospholipid Membranes. *Journal of Biological Chemistry*, *282*(22), 16644-16653. doi:10.1074/jbc.m701072200.

Nomikos, M., Sanders, J. R., Kashir, J., Sanusi, R., Buntwal, L., Love, D. & Lai, F. A. (2015). Functional disparity between human PAWP and PLCζ in the generation of Ca2+oscillations for oocyte activation. *Molecular Human Reproduction*, *21*(9), 702-710. doi:10.1093/molehr/gav034.

Nomikos, M., Sanders, J. R., Parthimos, D., Buntwal, L., Calver, B. L., Stamatiadis, P. & Lai, F. A. (2015). Essential Role of the EF-hand Domain in Targeting Sperm Phospholipase Cζ to Membrane Phosphatidylinositol 4,5-Bisphosphate (PIP2). *The Journal of biological chemistry*, *290*(49), 29519-29530. doi:10.1074/jbc.M115.658443.

Nomikos, M., Stamatiadis, P., Sanders, J. R., Beck, K., Calver, B. L., Buntwal, L. & Lai, F. A. (2017). Male infertility-linked point mutation reveals a vital binding role for the C2 domain of sperm PLCζ. *Biochemical Journal*, *474*(6), 1003-1016. doi:10.1042/bcj20161057.

Nomikos, M., Yu, Y., Elgmati, K., Theodoridou, M., Campbell, K., Vassilakopoulou, V. & Lai, F. A. (2013). Phospholipase Cζ rescues failed oocyte activation in a prototype of male factor infertility. *Fertility and sterility*, *99*(1), 76-85. doi:10.1016/j.fertnstert.2012.08.035.

Nordhoff, V., Fricke, R. K., Schüring, A. N., Zitzmann, M. & Kliesch, S. (2015). Treatment strategies for severe oligoasthenoteratozoospermia (OAT) (<0.1 million/mL) patients. *Andrology*, *3*(5), 856-863. doi:10.1111/andr.12077.

Norozi-Hafshejani, M., Tavalaee, M. & Nasr- Esfahani, M. H. (2019). Evaluation of comparison of clinical outcome treated oocyte with ionomycin and strontium chloride in infertile couple with previous failed *in vitro* fertilization. *Journal of Shahid Sadoughi University of Medical Sciences.* doi:10.18502/ssu.v27i2.1047.

Nowicka-Bauer, K., Ozgo, M., Lepczynski, A., Kamieniczna, M., Malcher, A., Skrzypczak, W. & Kurpisz, M. (2018). Human sperm proteins identified by 2-dimensional electrophoresis and mass spectrometry and their relevance to a transcriptomic analysis. *Reproductive Biology*, *18*(2), 151-160. doi:10.1016/j.repbio.2018.02.003.

Nozawa, K., Satouh, Y., Fujimoto, T., Oji, A. & Ikawa, M. (2018). Sperm-borne phospholipase C zeta-1 ensures monospermic fertilization in mice. *Scientific reports*, *8*(1), 1315-1315. doi:10.1038/s41598-018-19497-6.

Ogonuki, N., Inoue, K. & Ogura, A. (2011). Birth of Normal Mice Following Round Spermatid Injection Without Artificial Oocyte Activation. *Journal of Reproduction and Development*, *57*(4), 534-538. doi:10.1262/jrd.11-008m.

Ogura, A., Matsuda, J. & Yanagimachi, R. (1994). Birth of normal young after electrofusion of mouse oocytes with round spermatids. *Proceedings of the National Academy of Sciences of the United States of America*, *91*(16), 7460-7462. doi:10.1073/pnas.91.16.7460.

Osman, A., Alsomait, H., Seshadri, S., El-Toukhy, T. & Khalaf, Y. (2015). The effect of sperm DNA fragmentation on live birth rate after IVF or ICSI: a systematic review and meta-analysis. *Reproductive BioMedicine Online*, *30*(2), 120-127. doi:10.1016/j.rbmo.2014.10.018.

Palermo, G. (1992). Pregnancies after intracytoplasmic injection of single spermatozoon into an oocyte. *The Lancet*, *340*(8810), 17-18. doi:10.1016/0140-6736(92)92425-f.

Pan, Q., Ju, Z., Huang, J., Zhang, Y., Qi, C., Gao, Q. & Wang, C. (2013). PLCz functional haplotypes modulating promoter transcriptional activity are associated with semen quality traits in Chinese Holstein bulls. *PloS one*, *8*(3), e58795-e58795. doi:10.1371/journal.pone.0058795.

Pang, M. G. (1999). Detection of aneuploidy for chromosomes 4, 6, 7, 8, 9, 10, 11, 12, 13, 17, 18, 21, X and Y by fluorescence in-situ hybridization in spermatozoa from nine patients with oligoasthenoteratozoospermia undergoing intracytoplasmic sperm injection. *Human Reproduction*, *14*(5), 1266-1273. doi:10.1093/humrep/14.5.1266.

Park, J. H., Kim, S. K., Kim, J., Kim, J. H., Chang, J. H., Jee, B. C. & Kim, S. H. (2015). Relationship between phospholipase C zeta immunoreactivity and DNA fragmentation and oxidation in human sperm. *Obstetrics & gynecology science*, *58*(3), 232-238. doi:10.5468/ogs.2015.58.3.232.

Parrington, J. (2001). Does a soluble sperm factor trigger calcium release in the egg at fertilization? *J Androl*, *22*(1), 1-11.

Parrington, J., Davis, L. C., Galione, A. & Wessel, G. (2007). Flipping the switch: How a sperm activates the egg at fertilization.

Developmental Dynamics, *236*(8), 2027-2038. doi:10.1002/dvdy.21255.

Parrington, J., Swann, K., Shevchenko, V. I., Sesay, A. K. & Lai, F. A. (1996). Calcium oscillations in mammalian eggs triggered by a soluble sperm protein. *Nature*, *379*(6563), 364-368. doi:10.1038/379364a0.

Pelinck, M. J., Hoek, A., Simons, A. H. M., Heineman, M. J., van Echten-Arends, J. & Arts, E. G. J. M. (2010). Embryo quality and impact of specific embryo characteristics on ongoing implantation in unselected embryos derived from modified natural cycle *in vitro* fertilization. *Fertility and Sterility*, *94*(2), 527-534. doi:10.1016/j.fertnstert.2009.03.076.

Perry, A. C. F., Wakayama, T. & Yanagimachi, R. (1999). A Novel Trans-Complementation Assay Suggests Full Mammalian Oocyte Activation Is Coordinately Initiated by Multiple, Submembrane Sperm Components1. *Biology of Reproduction*, *60*(3), 747-755. doi:10.1095/biolreprod60.3.747.

Polanski, L. T., Baumgarten, M. N., Quenby, S., Brosens, J., Campbell, B. K. & Raine-Fenning, N. J. (2014). What exactly do we mean by 'recurrent implantation failure'? A systematic review and opinion. *Reproductive BioMedicine Online*, *28*(4), 409-423. doi:10.1016/j.rbmo.2013.12.006.

Pribenszky, C., Losonczi, E., Molnár, M., Lang, Z., Mátyás, S., Rajczy, K. & Vajta, G. (2010). Prediction of in-vitro developmental competence of early cleavage-stage mouse embryos with compact time-lapse equipment. *Reproductive BioMedicine Online*, *20*(3), 371-379. doi:10.1016/j.rbmo.2009.12.007.

Pribenszky, C., Nilselid, A. M. & Montag, M. (2017). Time-lapse culture with morphokinetic embryo selection improves pregnancy and live birth chances and reduces early pregnancy loss: a meta-analysis. *Reproductive BioMedicine Online*, *35*(5), 511-520. doi:10.1016/j.rbmo.2017.06.022.

Rahimizadeh, P., Topraggaleh, T. R., Nasr-Esfahani, M. H., Ziarati, N., Mirshahvaladi, S., Esmaeili, V. & Shahverdi, A. (2019). The alteration of PLCζ protein expression in unexplained infertile and asthenoteratozoospermic patients: A potential effect on sperm fertilization ability. *Molecular Reproduction and Development*, *87*(1), 115-123. doi:10.1002/mrd.23293.

Ramadan, W. M., Kashir, J., Jones, C. & Coward, K. (2012). Oocyte activation and phospholipase C zeta (PLCζ): diagnostic and therapeutic implications for assisted reproductive technology. *Cell communication and signaling: CCS*, *10*(1), 12-12. doi:10.1186/1478-811X-10-12.

Ramalho-Santos, J. (2011). A sperm's tail: the importance of getting it right. *Human Reproduction*, *26*(9), 2590-2591. doi:10.1093/humrep/der200.

Robinson, L., Gallos, I. D., Conner, S. J., Rajkhowa, M., Miller, D., Lewis, S. & Coomarasamy, A. (2012). The effect of sperm DNA fragmentation on miscarriage rates: a systematic review and meta-analysis. *Human Reproduction*, *27*(10), 2908-2917. doi:10.1093/humrep/des261.

Rogers, N. T., Hobson, E., Pickering, S., Lai, F. A., Braude, P. & Swann, K. (2004). Phospholipase Cζ causes Ca2+ oscillations and parthenogenetic activation of human oocytes. *Reproduction*, *128*(6), 697-702. doi:10.1530/rep.1.00484.

Rubino, P., Viganò, P., Luddi, A. & Piomboni, P. (2015). The ICSI procedure from past to future: a systematic review of the more controversial aspects. *Human Reproduction Update*, dmv050. doi:10.1093/humupd/dmv050.

Runft, L. L., Carroll, D. J., Gillett, J., Giusti, A. F., O'Neill, F. J. & Foltz, K. R. (2004). Identification of a starfish egg PLC-γ that regulates Ca2+ release at fertilization. *Developmental Biology*, *269*(1), 220-236. doi:10.1016/j.ydbio.2004.01.031.

Rutstein, S. O. & Shah, I. H. (2004). *Infecundity, Infertility, and Childlessness in DevelopingCountries*. Retrieved from Rybouchkin, A. V., Van der Straeten, F., Quatacker, J., De Sutter, P. & Dhont, M. (1997). Fertilization and pregnancy after assisted oocyte activation and intracytoplasmic sperm injection in a case of round-headed sperm associated with deficient oocyte activation capacity. *Fertil Steril*, *68*(6), 1144-1147. doi:10.1016/s0015-0282(97)00378-6.

Samanta, L., Agarwal, A., Swain, N., Sharma, R., Gopalan, B., Esteves, S. C. & Sabanegh, E. (2018). Proteomic Signatures of

Sperm Mitochondria in Varicocele: Clinical Use as Biomarkers of Varicocele Associated Infertility. *Journal of Urology*, *200*(2), 414-422. doi:10.1016/j.juro.2018.03.009.

Santella, L. & Dale, B. (2015). Assisted yes, but where do we draw the line? *Reproductive BioMedicine Online*, *31*(4), 476-478. doi:10.1016/j.rbmo.2015.06.013.

Sanusi, R., Yu, Y., Nomikos, M., Lai, F. A. & Swann, K. (2015). Rescue of failed oocyte activation after ICSI in a mouse model of male factor infertility by recombinant phospholipase Cζ. *Molecular human reproduction*, *21*(10), 783-791. doi:10.1093/molehr/gav042.

Saraswat, M., Joenväärä, S., Jain, T., Tomar, A. K., Sinha, A., Singh, S. & Renkonen, R. (2017). Human Spermatozoa Quantitative Proteomic Signature Classifies Normo- and Asthenozoospermia. *Molecular & cellular proteomics: MCP*, *16*(1), 57-72. doi:10.1074/mcp.M116.061028.

Saunders, C. M., Larman, M. G., Parrington, J., Cox, L. J., Royse, J., Blayney, L. M. & Lai, F. A. (2002). PLC zeta: a sperm-specific trigger of Ca(2+) oscillations in eggs and embryo development. *Development*, *129*(15), 3533-3544.

Schrimpf, R., Dierks, C., Martinsson, G., Sieme, H. & Distl, O. (2014). Genome-wide association study identifies phospholipase C zeta 1 (PLCz1) as a stallion fertility locus in Hanoverian warmblood horses. *PloS one*, *9*(10), e109675-e109675. doi:10.1371/journal.pone.0109675.

Sermondade, N., Hafhouf, E., Dupont, C., Bechoua, S., Palacios, C., Eustache, F. & Sifer, C. (2011). Successful childbirth after intracytoplasmic morphologically selected sperm injection without assisted oocyte activation in a patient with globozoospermia. *Human Reproduction*, *26*(11), 2944-2949. doi:10.1093/humrep/der258.

Sette, C., Bevilacqua, A., Geremia, R. & Rossi, P. (1998). Involvement of phospholipase Cgamma1 in mouse egg activation induced by a truncated form of the C-kit tyrosine kinase present in spermatozoa. *The Journal of cell biology*, *142*(4), 1063-1074. doi:10.1083/jcb.142.4.1063.

Sette, C., Paronetto, M. P., Barchi, M., Bevilacqua, A., Geremia, R. & Rossi, P. (2002). Tr-kit-induced resumption of the cell cycle in mouse eggs requires activation of a Src-like kinase. *The EMBO journal*, *21*(20), 5386-5395. doi:10.1093/emboj/cdf553.

Silber, S. J. & Johnson, L. (1998). Are spermatid injections of any clinical value? ROSNI and ROSI revisited. Round spermatid nucleus injection and round spermatid injection. *Human Reproduction*, *13*(3), 509-515. doi:10.1093/humrep/13.3.509.

Silber, S. J., Johnson, L., Verheyen, G. & Van Steirteghem, A. (2000). Round spermatid injection. *Fertility and Sterility*, *73*(5), 897-900. doi:10.1016/s0015-0282(00)00488-x.

Sinha, A., Singh, V., Singh, S. & Yadav, S. (2019). Proteomic analyses reveal lower expression of TEX40 and ATP6V0A2 proteins related to calcium ion entry and acrosomal acidification in asthenozoospermic males. *Life Sciences*, *218*, 81-88. doi:10.1016/j.lfs.2018.12.016.

Siva, A. B., Kameshwari, D. B., Singh, V., Pavani, K., Sundaram, C. S., Rangaraj, N. & Shivaji, S. (2010). Proteomics-based study on asthenozoospermia: differential expression of proteasome alpha complex. *MHR: Basic science of reproductive medicine*, *16*(7), 452-462. doi:10.1093/molehr/gaq009.

Sousa, M. & Tesarik, J. (1994). Fertiliza1tion and early embryology: Ultrastructural analysis of fertilization failure after intracytoplasmic sperm injection. *Human Reproduction*, *9*(12), 2374-2380. doi:10.1093/oxfordjournals.humrep.a138455.

Stitzel, M. L. & Seydoux, G. (2007). Regulation of the Oocyte-to-Zygote Transition. *Science*, *316*(5823), 407-408. doi:10.1126/science.1138236.

Stricker, S. A. (1997). Intracellular Injections of a Soluble Sperm Factor Trigger Calcium Oscillations and Meiotic Maturation in Unfertilized Oocytes of a Marine Worm. *Developmental Biology*, *186*(2), 185-201. doi:10.1006/dbio.1997.8594.

Stricker, S. A. (1999). Comparative Biology of Calcium Signaling during Fertilization and Egg Activation in Animals. *Developmental Biology*, *211*(2), 157-176. doi:10.1006/dbio.1999.9340.

Suh, P. G., Park, J. I., Manzoli, L., Cocco, L., Peak, J. C., Katan, M. & Ryu, S. H. (2008). Multiple roles of phosphoinositide-specific phospholipase C isozymes. *BMB Reports*, *41*(6), 415-434. doi:10.5483/bmbrep.2008.41.6.415.

Sutovsky, P., Manandhar, G., Wu, A. & Oko, R. (2003). Interactions of sperm perinuclear theca with the oocyte: Implications for oocyte activation, anti-polyspermy defense, and assisted reproduction. *Microscopy Research and Technique*, *61*(4), 362-378. doi:10.1002/jemt.10350.

Swann, K. (1990). A cytosolic sperm factor stimulates repetitive calcium increases and mimics fertilization in hamster eggs. *Development*, *110*(4), 1295-1302.

Swann, K. (1992). Different triggers for calcium oscillations in mouse eggs involve a ryanodine-sensitive calcium store. *The Biochemical journal*, *287 (Pt 1)*(Pt 1), 79-84. doi:10.1042/bj2870079.

Swann, K. & Lai, F. A. (2016). The sperm phospholipase C-ζ and Ca2+ signalling at fertilization in mammals. *Biochem Soc Trans*, *44*(1), 267-272. doi:10.1042/BST20150221.

Swann, K. & Ozil, J. P. (1994). Dynamics of the Calcium Signal That Triggers Mammalian Egg Activation. In *International Review of Cytology*. (pp. 183-222): Elsevier.

Swann, K., Saunders, C., Rogers, N. & Lai, F. (2006). PLCζ (zeta): A sperm protein that triggers Ca2+ oscillations and egg activation in mammals. *Seminars in Cell & Developmental Biology*, *17*(2), 264-273. doi:10.1016/j.semcdb.2006.03.009.

Swann, K. & Yu, Y. (2008). The dynamics of calcium oscillations that activate mammalian eggs. *The International Journal of Developmental Biology*, *52*(5-6), 585-594. doi:10.1387/ijdb.072530ks.

Tanaka, A., Nagayoshi, M., Takemoto, Y., Tanaka, I., Kusunoki, H., Watanabe, S. & Yanagimachi, R. (2015). Fourteen babies born after round spermatid injection into human oocytes. *Proceedings of the National Academy of Sciences of the United States of America*, *112*(47), 14629-14634. doi:10.1073/pnas.1517466112.

Tanaka, A., Suzuki, K., Nagayoshi, M., Tanaka, A., Takemoto, Y., Watanabe, S. & Yanagimachi, R. (2018). Ninety babies born after round spermatid injection into oocytes: survey of their development from fertilization to 2 years of age. *Fertility and Sterility*, *110*(3), 443-451. doi:10.1016/j.fertnstert.2018.04.033.

Tavalaee, M., Kiani-Esfahani, A. & Nasr-Esfahani, M. H. (2017). Relationship between phospholipase C-zeta, semen parameters, and chromatin status. *Systems Biology in Reproductive Medicine, 63*(4), 259-268. doi:10.1080/19396368.2017.1298006.

Tavalaee, M., Kiani-Esfahani, A. & Nasr-Esfahani, M. H. (2017). Relationship between Potential Sperm Factors Involved in Oocyte Activation and Sperm DNA Fragmentation with Intra-Cytoplasmic Sperm Injection Clinical Outcomes. *Cell J, 18*(4), 588-596. doi:10.22074/cellj.2016.4725.

Tavalaee, M., Nomikos, M., Lai, F. A. & Nasr-Esfahani, M. H. (2018). Expression of sperm PLCζ and clinical outcomes of ICSI-AOA in men affected by globozoospermia due to DPY19L2 deletion. *Reproductive BioMedicine Online, 36*(3), 348-355. doi:10.1016/j.rbmo.2017.12.013.

Tavalaee, M., Parivar, K., Shahverdi, A. H., Ghaedi, K. & Nasr-Esfahani, M. H. (2017). Status of sperm-born oocyte activating factors (PAWP, PLCζ) and sperm chromatin in uncapacitated, capacitated and acrosome-reacted conditions. *Human Fertility, 20*(2), 96-103. doi:10.1080/14647273.2016.1264011.

Taylor, S. L., Yoon, S. Y., Morshedi, M. S., Lacey, D. R., Jellerette, T., Fissore, R. A. & Oehninger, S. (2010). Complete globozoospermia associated with PLCζ deficiency treated with calcium ionophore and ICSI results in pregnancy. *Reproductive biomedicine online, 20*(4), 559-564. doi:10.1016/j.rbmo.2009.12.024.

The Practice Committee of ASRM. (2012). Intracytoplasmic sperm injection (ICSI) for non-male factor infertility: a committee opinion. *Fertil Steril, 98*(6), 1395-1399. doi:10.1016/j.fertnstert.2012.08.026.

Tejera, A., Mollá, M., Muriel, L., Remohí, J., Pellicer, A. & De Pablo, J. L. (2008). Successful pregnancy and childbirth after intracytoplasmic sperm injection with calcium ionophore oocyte activation in a globozoospermic patient. *Fertility and Sterility, 90*(4), 1202.e1201-1202.e1205. doi:10.1016/j.fertnstert.2007.11.056.

Tesarik, J. & Mendoza, C. (1996). Spermatid injection into human oocytes. I. Laboratory techniques and special features of zygote development. *Human Reproduction, 11*(4), 772-779. doi:10.1093/oxfordjournals.humrep.a019253.

Tesarik, J., Rolet, F., Brami, C., Sedbon, E., Thorel, J., Tibi, C. & Thebault, A. (1996). Spermatid injection into human oocytes. II. Clinical application in the treatment of infertility due to non obstructive azoospermia. *Human Reproduction*, *11*(4), 780-783. doi:10.1093/oxfordjournals.humrep.a019254.

Theodoridou, M., Nomikos, M., Parthimos, D., Gonzalez-Garcia, J. R., Elgmati, K., Calver, B. L. & Lai, F. A. (2013). Chimeras of sperm PLCζ reveal disparate protein domain functions in the generation of intracellular Ca2+ oscillations in mammalian eggs at fertilization. *Molecular human reproduction*, *19*(12), 852-864. doi:10.1093/molehr/gat070.

Torra-Massana, M., Cornet-Bartolomé, D., Barragán, M., Durban, M., Ferrer-Vaquer, A., Zambelli, F. & Vassena, R. (2019). Novel phospholipase C zeta 1 mutations associated with fertilization failures after ICSI. *Human Reproduction*, *34*(8), 1494-1504. doi:10.1093/humrep/dez094.

Van den Veyver, I. B. & Al-Hussaini, T. K. (2006). Biparental hydatidiform moles: a maternal effect mutation affecting imprinting in the offspring. *Human Reproduction Update*, *12*(3), 233-242. doi:10.1093/humupd/dmk005.

Vanderzwalmen, P., Zech, H., Birkenfeld, A., Yemini, M., Bertin, G., Lejeune, B. & Schoysman, R. (1997). Intracytoplasmic injection of spermatids retrieved from testicular tissue: influence of testicular pathology, type of selected spermatids and oocyte activation. *Human Reproduction*, *12*(6), 1203-1213. doi:10.1093/humrep/12.6.1203.

Verza, Jr. S. & Esteves, S. C. (2008). Sperm defect severity rather than sperm source is associated with lower fertilization rates after intracytoplasmic sperm injection. *International braz j urol*, *34*(1), 49-56. doi:10.1590/s1677-55382008000100008.

Virro, M. R., Larson-Cook, K. L. & Evenson, D. P. (2004). Sperm chromatin structure assay (scsa®) parameters are related to fertilization, blastocyst development, and ongoing pregnancy in *in vitro* fertilization and intracytoplasmic sperm injection cycles. *Fertility and Sterility*, *81*(5), 1289-1295. doi:10.1016/j.fertnstert.2003.09.063.

Whitaker, M. (2006). Calcium at fertilization and in early development. *Physiological reviews*, *86*(1), 25-88. doi:10.1152/ physrev.00023.2005.

WHO (Producer). (2010). *WHO laboratory manual for the examination and processing of human semen.*

Wong, C. C., Loewke, K. E., Bossert, N. L., Behr, B., De Jonge, C. J., Baer, T. M. & Pera, R. A. R. (2010). Non-invasive imaging of human embryos before embryonic genome activation predicts development to the blastocyst stage. *Nature Biotechnology*, *28*(10), 1115-1121. doi:10.1038/nbt.1686.

Wright, C., Milne, S. & Leeson, H. (2014). Sperm DNA damage caused by oxidative stress: modifiable clinical, lifestyle and nutritional factors in male infertility. *Reproductive BioMedicine Online*, *28*(6), 684-703. doi:10.1016/j.rbmo.2014.02.004.

Wu, A. T. H., Sutovsky, P., Manandhar, G., Xu, W., Katayama, M., Day, B. N. & Oko, R. (2007). PAWP, a Sperm-specific WW Domain-binding Protein, Promotes Meiotic Resumption and Pronuclear Development during Fertilization. *Journal of Biological Chemistry*, *282*(16), 12164-12175. doi:10.1074/jbc.m609132200.

Xu, Z., Williams, C. J., Kopf, G. S. & Schultz, R. M. (2003). Maturation-associated increase in IP3 receptor type 1: role in conferring increased IP3 sensitivity and Ca2+ oscillatory behavior in mouse eggs. *Developmental Biology*, *254*(2), 163-171. doi:10.1016/s0012-1606(02)00049-0.

Yamaguchi, T., Ito, M., Kuroda, K., Takeda, S. & Tanaka, A. (2017). The establishment of appropriate methods for egg-activation by human PLCZ1 RNA injection into human oocyte. *Cell Calcium*, *65*, 22-30. doi:10.1016/j.ceca.2017.03.002.

Yanagimachi, R., Wakayama, T., Kishikawa, H., Fimia, G. M., Monaco, L. & Sassone-Corsi, P. (2004). Production of fertile offspring from genetically infertile male mice. *Proceedings of the National Academy of Sciences of the United States of America*, *101*(6), 1691-1695. doi:10.1073/pnas.0307832100.

Yazawa, H. (2001). Oocyte activation and Ca2+ oscillation-inducing abilities of mouse round/elongated spermatids and the developmental capacities of embryos from spermatid injection. *Human Reproduction*, *16*(6), 1221-1228. doi:10.1093/humrep/16.6.1221.

Yazawa, H., Yanagida, K., Hayashi, S. & Sato, A. (2009). The oocyte activation and Ca2+ oscillation-inducing abilities of mouse and human dead (sonicated) spermatozoa. *Zygote*, *17*(2), 175-184. doi:10.1017/s0967199408005157.

Yin, X. & Eckberg, W. R. (2009). Characterization of phospholipases C β and γ and their possible roles inChaetopterusegg activation. *Molecular Reproduction and Development*, *76*(5), 460-470. doi:10.1002/mrd.20961.

Yoneda, A., Kashima, M., Yoshida, S., Terada, K., Nakagawa, S., Sakamoto, A. & Watanabe, T. (2006). Molecular cloning, testicular postnatal expression, and oocyte-activating potential of porcine phospholipase Cζ. *Reproduction*, *132*(3), 393-401. doi:10. 1530/rep.1.01018.

Yoon, S. Y., Jellerette, T., Salicioni, A. M., Lee, H. C., Yoo, M. S., Coward, K. & Fissore, R. A. (2008). Human sperm devoid of PLC, zeta 1 fail to induce Ca(2+) release and are unable to initiate the first step of embryo development. *The Journal of clinical investigation*, *118*(11), 3671-3681. doi:10.1172/JCI36942.

Young, C., Grasa, P., Coward, K., Davis, L. C. & Parrington, J. (2009). Phospholipase C zeta undergoes dynamic changes in its pattern of localization in sperm during capacitation and the acrosome reaction. *Fertility and Sterility*, *91*(5), 2230-2242. doi:10.1016/ j.fertnstert.2008.05.021.

Yu, Y., Saunders, C. M., Lai, F. A. & Swann, K. (2007). Preimplantation development of mouse oocytes activated by different levels of human phospholipase C zeta. *Human Reproduction*, *23*(2), 365-373. doi:10.1093/humrep/dem350.

Zhao, C., Huo, R., Wang, F. Q., Lin, M., Zhou, Z. M. & Sha, J. H. (2007). Identification of several proteins involved in regulation of sperm motility by proteomic analysis. *Fertility and Sterility*, *87*(2), 436-438. doi:10.1016/j.fertnstert.2006.06.057.

In: Intracytoplasmic Sperm Injection (ICSI) ISBN: 978-1-53619-762-4
Editor: Murid Javed

Chapter 5

Reconstruction of Zygote and Embryonic Development Following Microsurgical Restoration of the Diploid Constitution in the Human Tripronuclear Zygote

Abdul Munaf Sultan Ahamed*
Anova Fertility & Reproductive Health, Toronto, Canada

Abstract

Human cells have 46 chromosomes except the oocyte or sperm which has 23 chromosomes each. A normal fertilization is combination of 23 chromosomes from egg and 23 chromosomes from sperm to make a diploid zygote with 46 chromosomes. At fertilization each set of chromosomes can be viewed under the microscope as a pronucleus. During abnormal fertilization an extra (or more) set of 23 chromosomes (or pronucleus) is observed in the egg due to penetration of an egg by two or more sperm or by failure of the oocyte to extrude the second polar body. These

* Corresponding Author's E-mail: munafivf@gmail.com. EmbryoScience: www.embryo-science.com.

zygotes are abnormal as they contain more than 46 chromosomes. By micro-manipulation technique, extra set (s) of chromosomes can be aspirated from the oocyte to make this zygote contain only 46 chromosomes. This chapter describes such situations and explains procedure to reconstruct the zygote.

Keywords: pronuclei, 2PN, 3PN, abnormal fertilization, zygote, diploid

INTRODUCTION

The occurrence of triploidy in human oocytes fertilized through conventional IVF was about 1 to 5% (Kola et al., 1987; Rawlins et al., 1988). It can be as high as 30% (Balakier, 1993). Triploidy is a pathological state, the implantation results in early abortion or mid-trimester abortion. It may continue to term, which might result in alive or dead baby, usually retarded with internal and external deformity (Fryns et al., 1977; Chatterjee et al., 1983; Monrozies et al., 1986). Twenty per cent of aborted fetuses are known to be triploid (Boue et al., 1975).

Fertilization of human oocyte by a diploid sperm or non-extrusion of the first or second polar body (Malter and Cohen 1989) or polyspermy (Balakier, 1993) may result in triploidy. Polyspermic fertilizations may result from oocyte immaturity or over maturity, fractured or defective zona and incomplete or compromised cortical reaction (cited in: Balakier, 1993) but not associated with ovarian stimulation regimes or to age of patients (Diamond et al., 1985; Van Der Ven et al., 1985; Dandekar et al., 1990).

In the mouse, polyspermy can be corrected by microsurgery. Microsurgically restored tripronuclear (3PN) mouse zygotes to the diploid stage have been shown to be capable of surviving, resulting in the birth of normal live young (Feng and Gordon, 1996). A successful effort has been accomplished in microsurgical removal of a pronucleus from 3PN human zygotes (Kola et al., 1987; Malter and Cohen, 1989; Gordon et al., 1989).

Sufficient embryos are often available in assisted reproduction treatment procedures. Hence, the requirement to use 3PN embryos occurs occasionally. In the event of 3PN zygotes due to polyspermy could have serious implications for the patients in some particular cases where the number of oocytes collected is limited. In such situations microsurgical enucleation of a pronucleus (MEP) in 3PN zygotes may be helpful to the patient. For instant, enucleation of polyspermic zygotes could only be considered experimental and its safety remains to be elucidated. Therefore, the objective of the present investigation is to develop an effective technique for enucleation of a single pronucleus (PN) from 3PN zygotes and to determine the embryonic development *in vitro*.

MATERIALS AND METHODS

Human Spermatozoa Preparation

Husbands of female patients produced semen by masturbation. Spermatozoa preparation for insemination was done by the standard swim-up or density gradient centrifugation using Puresperm™ techniques in Medi-Cult™ culture medium. The spermatozoa preparation was incubated under a gaseous phase of 5% CO_2 in air at 37°C until use.

Ovarian Stimulation and Oocyte Retrieval

In order to achieve menstruation or down-regulation, subcutaneous injections of gonadotrophin releasing hormone agonist (Buserelin; Suprefact; Hoescht, Frankfurt, Germany) were commenced in the mid-luteal phase on the basis of blood estradiol, progesterone and LH levels that have reached baseline values and when the thickness of endometrium becomes 4mm or less. To initiate follicle recruitment, injections of follicle stimulating hormone (FSH; Metrodin; Serono, Rome, Italy) were administered for three days. Subsequently, to stimulate follicular development, human menopausal gonadotrophin (Pergonal 500; Serono, Rome, Italy) was administered according to the response of the patient. After achieving follicular size of 16mm or more, ovulation induction was performed with an injection of a 10,000 IU of human chorionic gonadotrophin (hCG; Pregnyl; Organon, Oss, Holland). Oocyte retrieval (OR) was carried out by ultrasound guided vaginal aspiration about 36h post hCG injection.

Insemination and Culture Techniques

In Vitro Fertilization (IVF)

Oocytes were inseminated individually in 200 ul micro-droplets of equilibrated Medi-Cult™ culture medium under embryo-tested mineral oil (M8410, Sigma Chemicals, USA) previously adjusted to contain 100,000/mL motile spermatozoa. The inseminated oocytes were cultured in an atmosphere of 5% CO_2 in air at 37°C. The oocytes were denuded 18-22h later with denuding pipettes (ART No. 1670, International Medical Products BV, Zutphen, Holland).

Determination of Fertilization

Fertilization was set 18h to 20h after IVF. The oocytes were considered fertilized when two distinct pronuclei (2PN; diploid) and two polar bodies (PBs) were visible (**Figure 1**). Zygotes with three or more PNs are considered polyspemic if 2PBs are present. 3PN (3PN) and other polyspermic (>3PN) zygotes were cultured separately.

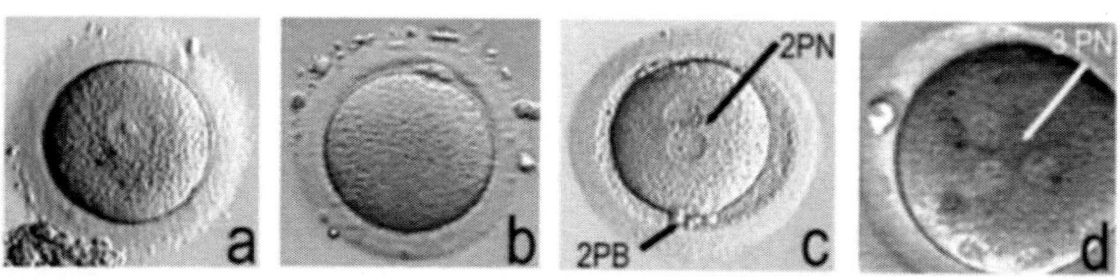

Figure 1. Pictures of different developmental stages of oocytes and signs of normal fertilization. (a) Immature oocyte, also called GV; (b) A mature oocyte at metaphase 2 (c) normal fertilization showing 2 PN and 2 PBs and (d) Abnormal fertilization showing 3 PN.

Ultra Micro-Droplet (UMD) Culture

Zygotes were cultured in ultra micro-droplet (UMD) cultures of equilibrated Medi-Cult™ medium under mineral oil in an atmosphere of 5% CO_2 in air at 37°C as previously described (Ali et al., 2000; Ali et al., 2002). Concisely, UMDs were in the order of 1.5 to 2uL of culture medium for culturing 3 to 9 human embryos. These were formed using a finely drawn out Pasteur pipette in culture dishes previously filled with equilibrated mineral oil. The dishes were incubated under a gaseous phase of 5% CO_2 in air at 37°C. The medium was not replaced on a daily basis. Cleavage and embryo quality was assessed about 48h post-insemination. Excess normal embryos (diploid) were frozen-stored following embryo transfer. 3PN embryos were cultured separately in UMD prior to and after microsurgical removal of a single PN up to day 5/6. Cleavage and embryo quality of enucleated 3PN embryos were performed on a daily basis.

The extreme low volume employed was to prevent dilution of autocrine and paracrine factors (APFs) released by the embryos which in turn improves the quality and viability of the embryos (Paria and Dey, 1990; Paria et al., 1991; Canesco et al., 1992; Almagor et al., 1996). In fact, a separate study has shown that the clinical pregnancy rate from day 2 embryos generated in continuous UMD (cUMD) cultures for 48hrs in MediCult™ medium following ICSI was about 62% (41/66) (Ali et al., 2002). This observation implies the possible involvement of APFs in the generation of quality embryos and hence illustrates the usefulness of the UMD culture procedure.

Determination of Embryo Quality

The quality of human day 2 embryos was determined as described previously. The parameters employed to determine the efficacy of MEP procedures are: (i) zygote developmental arrest rate, (ii) average blastomere number, (iii) average embryo grade, (iv) proportion of embryos that progressed to 4-cell stage and above on day 2, (v) proportion of embryos that attained an embryo grade of three and above in a score ranging from 4 to 1 (Ali et al., 2000; Ali et al., 2002), (vi) Daily development of MEP embryos compared to previous reports. Since most healthy day 2 human embryos generally attain the 4-cell stage, an average blastomere score (ABN) of 4 and above is considered excellent in a range of 2 to 6. The embryos are graded (average embryo grade; AEG) according to a scale of 1 to 4, where the numerical 1 denoted poor quality, and 4, excellent quality. Three laboratory personnel graded embryos collectively to avoid bias with the use of a television monitor.

Technique for Measuring Size of Pronuclei

To measure the size of the pronuclei, an improvised image analysis technique (Ali et al., 2002) is employed. The diameter of the PN is measured on the image of the zygote on the TV monitor screen. Two to three laboratory personnel measured the diameter of the pronuclei collectively to avoid bias. Initially, the diameter of the PN closest to the polar bodies is recorded later on the PN or pronuclei distal to the polar bodies are noted.

Microsurgical Enucleation of PN (MEP)

Using an ICSI holding pipette, the 3PN zygote is held by suction at the 9 o'clock position and located in such a way that all 3PNs are distinctly and clearly visible with the polar bodies oriented at the 12 or 6 o'clock positions. The objective of this exercise is to micro-surgically remove a single PN that is distal to the polar bodies from zygotes generated after conventional IVF. The PN which is remote from the polar bodies and is larger or largest (Rawlins et al., 1988; Malter and Cohen, 1989) is most likely derived from the sperm. The PN that has been recognized to be removed is brought into focus. The nuclear membrane of the target PN should be distinctly and clearly visible. At the 3 o'clock position parallel to the holding pipette, an ICSI injection needle is brought into focus. The injection pipette is then injected partially into the zygote but short of touching the PNs. The membrane of the zygote is sucked gently into the injection pipette until it breaks. The injection pipette is then positioned into contact with the target PN which is then sucked into the pipette very gently until the entire PN is inside the injection pipette. This method may, sometimes, destroy the target PN, particularly if the internal diameter of the injection pipette is 7µ. The micro-surgically mended zygote which now has 2PNs is later cultured by standard techniques.

Culture Media

Embryo culture medium from Medi-Cult™ (Medi-Cult a/s, Lerso Parkalle 42, Copenhagen 2100, Denmark) was used for sperm preparation, insemination, embryo culture and embryo transfer.

Incidence of Polyspermy

The incidence of polyspermy was determined by retrospective analysis of data.

Diameter of Pronuclei of Normal Diploid Zygotes

The diameter of the PNs of probably normal diploid zygotes was measured as described earlier in this communication. A total of 20 diploid zygotes were examined.

Specific Experiments

Experiment 1

The MEP-derived zygotes and normal (2PN) sibling human oocytes were cultured in UMD in the Medi-Cult™ medium. On a daily basis, succeeding progress of the MEP zygotes was recorded until the growing discontinued. Only 2PN embryos were cultured up to day 2 cleaved stages. Following embryo transfer, excess normal day 2 embryos were frozen-stored. On day 2, the attribute of the day 2 embryos in the MEP and normal embryos were correlated as formerly described (Ali et al., 2000; Ali 2003).

Experiment 2

Using the cUMD IVM technique (Ali, 2003), discarded GV-stage oocytes were matured *in vitro*. These oocytes were injected with 5 sperm obtained from respective husbands by standard ICSI procedures. Subsequently, the diameters of the pronuclei were measured using the image of the zygote on a TV screen by at least two or more personnel to avoid bias. To facilitate measurement of diameter of the pronuclei, a glass measuring grid was fixed on the microscope, directed and superimposed on the TV screen. The images were duplicated with permanent ink by drawing over the image of the grids that appear on the screen. Using an oocyte holding pipette, the zygote were immobilized and located for measurement. The PN to be measured was placed and aligned over the grid markings on the TV screen. Measurements of specific pronuclei and their relevant location from the polar body were then recorded.

Statistical Analysis

Statistical analyses were performed with the paired t-test, 2-sample t-test, or two by two tables as suitable. A value of $p < 0.05$ was considered statistically significant.

Results

Incidence of Polyspermy

For 912 eggs retrieved, the occurrence of polyspermy was about 7 to 8% but increased to nearly 20% out of 358 eggs in patients that had polyspermy (Table 1).

Table 1. Incidence of unipronuclear, normal, tripronuclear and polyspermic zygotes in conventional IVF procedure. The values are number (%)

Description	0PN	1PN	2PN	3PN	>3PN	Total Fertilized
Overall (n = 912)	177 (19.4)	12 (1.3)	652 (71.5)	64 (7.0)	7 (0.8)	735 (80.6)
Cases with ≥3PN (n = 358)	94 (26.3)	8 (2.2)	185 (51.7)	64 (17.9)	7 (2.0)	264 (73.7)

Table 2. Characteristics of pronuclei of apparently normal diploid zygotes

Description/PN Diameter	**PN Closest to PB**	**PN Distal to PB**
Mean Diameter (SE)	19.1μ (0.261)	22.1μ (0.206)*
Median Diameter	19μ	22μ
Range	18.6-20.0μ	21.7-23.0μ
n	21	21
Diameter Frequency distribution, n (%)		
15μ	1 (4.8%)	0
18μ	3 (14.3%)	0
19μ	7 (33.3%)	0
20μ	10 (47.6%)	2 (9.5%)
21μ	0	2 (9.5%)
22μ	0	9 (42.9%)
23μ	0	8 (38.1%)

Diameter of Pronuclei of Normal Diploid Zygotes

In 20 normal diploid zygotes the mean diameter of PN closest and distal to the PB was 19.1μ and 22.1μ respectively (Table 2). Paired t-test disclosed these two values to be statistically highly significantly distinct ($p = 0.0000$). The diameters of individual PNs in diploid zygotes are not alike. The PN closest to the PB is always smaller than the distal PN.

Experiment 1

The developmental efficiency of the 26 MEP embryos appears to be similar to that reported by Balakier (Balakier, 1993) for 3PN embryos or vitrified 3PN or fresh normal 2PN embryos (Ali et al., 1996). Not less than 92% of the MEP embryos went through two cell cycles, 69% cavitated and 17% progressed to the blastocyst stage (Table 3). The embryo quality of day 2 MEP and normal embryos were very nearly indistinguishable in all regards (Table 4).

Table 3. Development of Microsurgically Corrected 3PN, Sibling and Non-sibling 2PN and vitrified 3PN Zygotes. The values are No. (Cleavage %)

Developmental Stage	3PN (Enucleated)	2PN (Sibling)	2PN (Non-Sib)	3PN (Vitrified) (Ali, 1996)
1-cell	26	45	652	15
2 to 4-cell	24 (92%)	42 (93.3%)*	640 (98.2%)*	14 (93.3%)
8-to 16-cell	24 (92%)	-	-	12 (80.0%)
16-to 32 cell	18 (69%)	-	-	5 (33.3%)
Early cavitation	5 (17%)	-	-	0
Blastocyst	0	-	-	-

* Embryos originating from these 2PN were transferred and excess embryos frozen on day 2 after ET.

Table 4. Embryo Quality of Microsurgically Corrected 3PN and 2PN Embryos at the Day 2 Cleaved Stages

Description	Average Blastomere Number (1SD)	Average Embryo Grade (1SD)	% > 4 Blastomeres	% > Grade 3	No. of Embryos
2PN	3.3 (0.8906)	3.2 (0.7485)	58.6%	75.9%	29
3PN (Enucleated)	3.3 (0.9441)	3.2 (0.8165)	58.3%	70.8	24
Significance	p = 0.3806	p = 0.3274	p = 1.000	p = 0.9200	

In a separate study, following conventional IVF the diameters of individual PN of 20 triploid zygotes generated was also determined. One PN closest to the PB was always of smaller (diameter 16.8μ) while the remaining two PNs distal the polar were of similar sizes (19.6μ and 19.7μ p = 7157) but statistically significantly (p = 0.0000) larger than that closest to PB (Table 5).

Table 5. Characteristics of pronuclei of tripronuclear zygotes generated in conventional IVF

Description/PN Diameter	**PN Closest to PB**	**PN Closest to PB$^{+\#}$**	
		PN1	PN2
Mean Diameter (SE)	16.8µ (0.6175)	19.6µ (0.665)	19.7µ (0.6893)
Median Diameter	18µ	21µ	20µ
Range	12.0-20.0µ	14.0-22.0µ	14.0-23.0µ
n	20	20	20

$^{+}$ Significantly different from PN closest to PB ($p = 0.000$).

$^{\#}$ PN1 and PN2 are statistically similar ($p = 0.7157$).

Experiment 2

This experiment proposed to measure the diameters of pronuclei of 11 cUMD-IVM oocytes. Even though 5 spermatozoa were injected into each IVM egg, the number of PNs formed was not identical in all eggs.

Table 6. The diameters of individual pronuclei generated in *in vitro* matured human oocytes after injection with 5 spermatozoa

Zygote no.	**PN closest to PB**	**PN distal to PB****			
	PN 1	PN 2	PN 3	PN4	PN5
1	17.1	22	22	21	-
2	17.5	20	20	20	-
3	16	20	20	21	22
4	19	20	20	22	-
5	12	14	15	-	-
6	13	15	15	-	-
7	12	15	15	-	-
8	13	15	15	-	-
9	13	15	15	-	-
10	20	22	22	-	-
11	17	22	20	22	-
Mean (SE)	15.4 (0.8777)	18.2 (1.007)	18.1 (0.919)	21.2 (0.3742)	22

** The maximum number of PNs formed after injection of 5 spermatozoa is 5 (one from egg and four from spermatozoa). All values are in microns (µ). Values for diameter of PN contributed by the egg is statistically significantly different to those of PNs contributed by the sperm ($p = 0.0000$). The diameters of PNs contributed by sperm were statistically similar.

All 11 eggs exhibited at least 3PNs, 5 eggs exhibited 4PNs and 1 egg exhibited 5PNs, none exhibited 6PNs. The PN diameters/sizes of the 11 individual eggs injected with 5 spermatozoa is given in Table 6. The mean diameters of individual PNs were as follows: PN contributed by the egg was ~15.4µ, and that contributed by the sperms (PNs distal to the PB) to be ~18.2µ, ~18.1µ, ~21.2µ and 22.0µ (the mean of all PNs distal to the PB was 18.8µ). Paired t test between the PNs closest and distal to PBs of zygotes representing equal numbers of PNs contributed by the egg and sperms revealed a highly significant difference between PNs contributed by the egg and that contributed by the sperms ($p = 0.000$, $n = 11$). Paired t tests between diameters of PNs contributed by sperm showed statistically non significant difference ($p = 0.6761$, $n = 11$).

Discussion

In human IVF procedures, 3PN zygotes are a common existence. In the authors' laboratory, the frequency of polyspermy is in the order of 7 to 8% in all patients that have gone through IVF treatment in the course of the stated period but the occurence is higher (19-20%) only if patients with polyspermy were calculated distinctly. This breakthrough supports the presumption that some patients are apparently more prone to polyspermy than others and this is probably related to defects in the oocyte such as immaturity or over maturity, fractured or defective zona and incomplete or compromised cortical reaction (cited in: Balakier (Balakier, 1993)).

The majority of women produce many eggs and accordingly the loss of about 7 to 8% of the eggs to polyspermy may not compromise their chances for embryo transfer. Nevertheless, polyspermy could be disadvantageous if only few eggs were available. In such situations, MEP of the affected zygotes could restore the pronuclei constitution of the zygote to the diploid or normal stage. The doubt that arises is whether or not MEP is completely safe. In animal studies, Feng and Gordon (Dandekar et al., 1990), have shown MEP to have no deleterious effect on the genetical constitution of mice derived from MEP-treated mouse embryos. Mice derived from the MEP experiment seemed apparently normal. MEP-derived mice later reproduced normally.

Former attempts at MEP in human 3PN zygotes were not very successful. Zygotes either did not survive the MEP procedure or the proportion of zygotes that survived and subsequently underwent cleavage was limited (Rawlins, 1988; Malter and Cohen 1989; Gordon et al., 1989). Some of the difficulties faced were the recognition of the male pronuclei. The general criteria adopted to recognize the male pronuclei were (i) increased size of male pronuclei, (ii) pronuclei with remnant sperm tail (iii) greater distance from polar body. Earlier workers report complication in identifying the male pronuclei. The sperm-tail is usually not seen and the sizes of the pronuclei appear similar. The third criterion of relative distance from polar body was applied to classify the male pronuclei for MEP.

The PN contributed by the sperm, inappropriately called the male PN, is thought to be larger than the PN contributed by the egg. To illustrate this point a small number of discarded human GV oocytes were matured *in vitro* and consequently injected each egg with five sperms contributed by their respective husbands of the donors of the GV eggs. Following day, the sizes or more appropriately, the diameters of the pronuclei were measured. Former workers faced the difficulty of precisely measuring the sizes of the PN. Therefore, the accidental removal of the pronuclei contributed by the egg would have resulted in diandrogenic zygotes. However in the existing study we have devised an improvised image analysis technique to measure the size of the PN somewhat accurately. Interestingly, in 21 apparently normal diploid zygotes, a single PN closest to the polar body appeared smaller (~19μ) in diameter while all other pronuclei were slightly larger (~22μ). Likewise in 20 triploid zygotes generated by conventional IVF, the PN closest to the PB was also found to be smaller (diameter 16.8μ) than the two remaining PNs distal the PB were of similar sizes (19.6μ and 19.7μ; $p = 7157$) but statistically significantly ($p = 0.0000$) larger than that closest to PB.

In IVM eggs the injection of 5 spermatozoa resulted in a similar finding of one small PN close to the PB and the remaining PNs distal to the PB were larger. All larger PNs in a particular polyspermic zygote were statistically similar. Therefore it is reasonable to speculate that the

PN contributed by the sperm is larger than that of the egg. Another finding of interest is that the mean sizes of PNs appear to become progressively smaller as the numbers of PNs increases in the zygotes, e.g.: the mean diameter of the PN contributed by the egg decreased from 19.1μ; 16.8μ and 15.4μ in 2PN, 3PN and >3PN zygotes respectively (Tables 2, 5, 6). A related trend is not clearly observable with PNs contributed by the sperm.

One more factor that may have contributed to the less than optimal survival in preceding reports was probably related to the enucleation technique and size of enucleation pipette used. In contrast however, in the present study 92% of all MEP zygotes progressed through at least two cleavage cycles (i.e., day 2 and 3 stages), 69% progressed to the late morula and partial compacted morula stages (day 4 stages) and 17% cavitated but were of poor quality when cultured in Medi-Cult™ medium. The improved survival following MEP in the present study compared to previous studies could be related to the fine and elegant technique employed and the size of the enucleation pipette used. The enucleation pipette used was the ICSI pipette with about 7-9μ (ID-OD respectively) in diameter. The smaller enucleation pipette used may have contributed to better survival as the trauma to the zygote would have been less.

In the present study, the *in vitro* development exhibited by the MEP zygotes is similar to or improved than that reported by Balakier (1993) for 3PN human embryos, or vitrified unipronuclear and 3PN embryos, and normal 2PN embryos (Ali, 1996) when cultured under moderately similar conditions. Most MEP embryos (92%) underwent day 2 and 3 cleavage cycles, 69% progressed to the late morula or compacted morula stage and 17% cavitated. These cleavage cycles are reminiscent of the developmental potential of normal diploid embryos. It is likely that MEP employed in the present study may have restored the triploid embryo to its normal genetic constitution. Furthermore the embryo quality in day 2 MEP zygotes and normal 2PN embryos appear to be statistically similar (Table 3). These findings indicate that the MEP procedure employed in the present study had no detrimental impact whatsoever on the survival and viability of the enucleated 3PN zygote.

It remains to be seen whether the MEP embryos generated by the technique employed in the investigation are completely safe and genetically normal in all respects. Despite studies in the mouse indicate MEP embryos can give rise to normal young it is however essential that the safety of such embryos be ascertained prior to human application. Preimplantation genetic diagnosis and other molecular genetics methods could be applied to ascertain the safety of MEP embryos in human assisted reproduction treatment procedures.

In addition to its application in human assisted reproduction procedures, MEP may have other applications in cell biology research. The enucleated PN and the MEP embryo could be used for other experiments to advance our understanding of the cellular processes involved in syngamy, cell division, gene expression, imprinting, effect of PN transfer, gamete manipulation, etc.

Conclusion

In conclusion, an effective and non-traumatic method of removal of a single PN from a 3PN embryo has been developed. Even though animal studies have shown MEP embryos to be normal, it can be applied in human assisted reproduction treatment after questions referring to safety have been demonstrated. This technique could also be useful in experimental biology.

Disclaimer

Anova Fertility & Reproductive Health, Toronto, Canada are not involved in this study.

References

[1] Kola, I., Trounson, A., Dawson, G., Rogers, P. (1987) Tripronuclear human oocytes: altered cleavge patterns and subsequent karotypic analysis of embryos. *Biol. Reprod.* 37:395.

[2] Rawlins, R. G., Binor, Z., Radwanska, E. and Dmowski, W. P. (1988). Microsurgical enucleation of tripronuclear human zygotes. *Fertil. Steril.* 50: 266-272.
[3] Balakier, H. (1993): Tripronuclear human zygotes: the first cell cycle and subsequent development. *Hum. Repro.* 8: 1892-1897.
[4] Fryns, J. P., van de Kerchkhove, A., Goddeeris, P., van der Berghe, H. (1977) Unusually long survival in a case of full triploidy of meternal origin. *Hum. Genet.* 38: 147.
[5] Chatterjee, M. S., Tajani, N. A., Verma, U. L., Weiss, R. R. (1983) Prenatal diagnosis of triploidy. *Int. J. Gynaecol. Obst.* 21: 155-157.
[6] Monrozies, X., Monrozies, M., Parinaud, J., Berrebi, A. (1986) La triploidie. *J. Gynecol. Obst. Biol. Reprod. Paris* 15: 893-900.
[7] Boue, J., Boue, A., Lazer, P. The epidemiology of human spontaneous abortion with chromosomal anomalies. In: *Aging Gametes, Their Biology and Pathology*, Edited by RJ Blandau. Basel, Karger, 1975, p 330.
[8] Malter, H. E. and Cohen, J. (1989) Partial zona dissection of the human oocyte: a nontraumatic method using micromanipulation to assist zona pellucida penetration. *Fertil. Steril.* 51: 139.
[9] Diamond, M. P., Rogers, J. B., Webster, B. W., Vaughn, W. K. and Wentz, A. C. (1985) Polyspermy: effect of varying stimulation protocols and inseminating sperm concentrations. *Fertil. Steril.*, 43, 777-780.
[10] Van Der Ven, H. H., Al Hassani, S., Diedrich, k., Hamerich, U., Lehmann, F. and Krebs, D. (1985) Polyspermy in *in vitro* fertilization of human oocytes: frequency and possible causes. *Ann. N. Y. Acad. Sci.*, 442, 88-95.
[11] Dandekar, M. P., Martin, M. C. and Glass, R. H. (1990) Polynuclear embryos after *in vitro* fertilization. *Fertil. Steril.*, 53, 510-514.
[12] Feng, Y. L. and Gordon, J. W. (1996) Birth of normal mice after removal of the supernumerary male pronucleus from polyspermic zygotes. *Hum. Repro.* vol 11, no. 2 pp. 341-344.
[13] Gordon, J. W., Grunfeld, L., Garrisi, G. J., Navot, D. and Laufer, N. (1989) Successful microsurgical removal of a pronucleus from tripronuclear human zygotes. *Fertil. Steril.* 52: 367-372.

[14] Ali, J., AlNatsha, S. D. and Shahata, M. A. M. (2000) Formulation of a protein-free medium for human assisted reproduction. *Human Reprod.* 15(1): 145-156.
[15] Ali, J., Rahbar, S., Burjaq, H., Sultan, AM., Al Flamerzi, M., Shahata, MAM. (2002) Ultra Micro-Environment Culture and Routine Laser Assisted Hatching Procedures Significantly Increase Clinical Pregnancy Rates. *Proceedings of the 21st Annual Scientific Meeting of the Fertility Society of Australia* (Abtr.), 23-26 Oct 2002, Gold Coast, Australia (abtr).
[16] Paria, B. C. and Dey, S. K. (1990) Preimplantation embryo development *in vitro*: cooperative interaction amonmg embryos and role of growth factors. *Proc. Natl. Acad. Sci. USA* 87:4756-4760.
[17] Paria, B. C. Tsukamura, H. and Dey, S. K. (1991) Epidermal growth factor specific protein tyrosine phosphorylation in preimplantation embryo development. *Biol. Reprod.* 45:711-718.
[18] Canesco, R. S., Sparks, A. E., Pearson, R. E. et al. (1992) Embryo density and medium volume effects on early murine embryo development. *J. Assist. Reprod. Genet.* 9:454-457.
[19] Almagor, M., Bejar, C., Kafka, I. et al. (1996) Pregnancy rates after communal growth of preimplantation of human embryos *in vitro*. *Fertil. Steril.* 66:394-397.
[20] Ali, J. (2003) *A Practical Guide to Mouse Preimplantation Embryology and Human Assisted Reproduction Technology*. JN Shelton, Ed. Ladybrook Publishers, Perth, Australia, ISBN 0-75411-647-6.
[21] Ali, J. (1996) Developmental competence of unipronuclear and triploid day-2 human embryos after vitrification with VS14. *Med. Sci. Res.* (UK) 24:377-378.

In: Intracytoplasmic Sperm Injection (ICSI) ISBN: 978-1-53619-762-4
Editor: Murid Javed

Chapter 6

ASSISTED REPRODUCTIVE TECHNOLOGY OUTCOME BEFORE AND AFTER VARICOCELE REPAIR

Hamed Al Ali*[1], *MD and Naif Al Hathal*[2,*], *MD
[1]Department of Urology, King Fahad Specialist Hospital, Dammam, Saudi Arabia
[2]Department of Urology, King Faisal Specialist Hospital and Research Center, Riyadh, Saudi Arabia

ABSTRACT

The varicocele is a dilated vein of pampiniform plexus. It could be clinical or subclinical. It is a common cause of male infertility with a prevalence rate of 15% in normal adult, 30% in men with primary infertility, and 80% in men with secondary infertility. It is more common on the left side. The varicocele deteriorates sperm quality due to testicular hyperthermia, testicular hypoxia, hormonal disturbances, apoptosis, increased reactive oxygen species, increased sperm DNA fragmentation and back flow of toxic metabolites. Several nonsurgical and surgical approaches have been advocated. The best outcome has been reported after

* Corresponding Author's E-mail: alnaif@yahoo.com.

microsurgical repair. The varicocele repair can increase rate of spontaneous pregnancy, and increase in pregnancy and live birth rate if performed prior to ART.

Keywords: varicocele, male infertility, sperm DNA fragmentation, testicular hyperthermia, testicular hypoxia, sperm damage

INTRODUCTION

Testis has a special composition of venous drainage system in a form of network that allows the process of heat exchange; Known as pampiniform plexus veins (Setchell and Brooks 1988). Varicocele is a dilated, elongated, and tortuous vein of pampiniform plexus, which is likely related to intravenous valvular incompetence that allows blood reflux into spermatic vein (Hamada, Esteves, and Agarwal 2013; Miyaoka and Esteves 2012). It has been divided into clinical and sub-clinical varicocele. The clinical varicocele is detected by physical examination and classified into three grades. The grade III varicocele is visible and palpable at rest, grade II is palpable at rest and grade I is palpable during valsalva manoeuver. The subclinical varicocele cannot be detected clinically. It has to be diagnosed by Doppler ultrasound (Miyaoka and Esteves 2012; Baigorri and Dixon 2016).

The varicocele is considered as a common cause of infertility with a prevalence rate of 15% in normal adult, 30% in male with primary infertility, and 80% in male with secondary infertility (Alsaikhan et al. 2016). It is more common on the left side and observed in 78% to 93% of cases, while only 2% of patients present with right-side varicocele. The bilateral varicocele is observed in 84% of the cases (Lipshultz and Niederberger 2009; Gat et al. 2006).

There are several hypotheses proposing the mechanism by which a varicocele may exert a deleterious effect on spermatogenesis and fertility potential. These include; scrotal hyperthermia, oxidative stress (OS), deoxyribonucleic acid (DNA) fragmentation, apoptosis, hormonal disturbances, testicular hypoperfusion, testicular hypoxia, and backflow of toxic metabolites (El-Domyati et al. 2010; Agarwal et al. 2016). Different methods have been developed for varicocelectomy or varicocele repair including varicocele embolization, laparoscopic repair, and surgical ligation with or without microscope in the retroperitoneum, inguinal canal or subinguinally (Al Bakri et al. 2012). Varicocele repair can significantly improve semen parameters in 60% to 80% of men, and 20% to 60% improvement in achieving spontaneous pregnancy (Marmar et al. 2007). There is significant improvement in pregnancy and live birth rates in men undergoing varicocele repair before assisted reproductive technology (ART) (Kim et al. 2013; Kirby 2016).

ETIOLOGY

The venous drainage system of the testis originates from small parenchymal veins which drain either into groups of veins near the mediastinum testis, or veins on the surface of the testis, that anastomose together to form a network of testicular veins surrounding the testicular artery known as pampiniform plexus. The pampiniform plexus veins will join at the level of inguinal canal to from two to three veins which then become bilaterally a single spermatic vein that ascend to drain into the inferior vena cava from the right side and to renal vein from the left side. Left testicular vein is longer than counterpart by 8–10 cm, and it runs vertically to drain into the left renal vein at a right angle unlike the right testicular vein, that run obliquely to drain directly into the inferior vena cava. This anatomical variation will increase the hydrostatic pressure of left testicular vein predisposing it to venous valve incompetence and spermatic cord vein dilation.

The left side varicocele is observed in 78% to 93% of cases, while only 2% of patients present with isolated right-side varicocele, that can be associated and brought into concern in cases of retroperitoneal or pelvic pathology (Lipshultz and Niederberger 2009; Gat et al. 2006). On the other hand bilateral varicocele can be observed in 84% of cases (Gat et al. 2006). Although it has been reported that absence of valve can be a significant cause of varicocele, other investigations reported 26.6% of men presenting with varicocele had competent valve (Sofikitis et al. 1993; Braedel et al. 1994). Other etiologies mentioned in the literature include; reflux of left adrenal gland catecholamines that lead to left testicular vein contraction, and a rare condition such as nutcracker syndrome (Comhaire and Vermeulen 1974; Braedel et al. 1994). The etiology of varicocele is still an area of interest that needs further investigation.

PATHOPHYSIOLOGY

Hyperthermia

Normal spermatogenesis process needs an optimal testicular temperature which is less than core body temperature by 2.5 °C. Testicular insult by hyperthermia due to varicocele can impair this process. This is widely accepted hypothesis that is supported by evidence. Varicocele can increase scrotal temperature by refluxing warm abdominal blood to pampiniform plexus through incompetent valves of spermatic and cremasteric veins. This will result in decreasing testosterone levels, Sertoli cell, and Leydig cell secretory function (Rajfer et al. 1987; Sofikitis and Miyagawa 1992; Khera and Lipshultz 2008). The relation between heat exposure and reactive oxygen species (ROS) generation has been demonstrated in several studies. Heat stress can increase the production of ROS from plasma membrane, mitochondria, cytoplasm, and peroxisome (Morgan et al. 2003; Ikeda et al. 1999). Also heat stress can enhance the production of nitric oxide (NO) and nitric oxide synthase (NOS) that can adversely affect sperm motility and lead to sperm apoptosis (Rosselli et al. 1995)22. Scrotal hyperthermia can produce ROS in other possible processes including insufficient heat shock proteins, and increased activity of xanthine oxidase (Yeşilli et al. 2005; Mitropoulos 1996).

Testicular Hypoxia

Varicocele association with hypoxia and infertility attract the researchers to focus on this correlation. High internal spermatic venous pressure that exceeds testicular arteriolar pressure can lead to testicular tissue ischemia, which had been proved by histological evaluation. Hypoxia inducible factor 1 (HIF-1) mediates the response of ischemic tissue to hypoxia, mainly determined by HIF-1 Alpha subunit, that is present in high level in the internal spermatic vein of infertile men with varicocele (Lee, Jeng, and Lee 2006). Also, this ischemic change will induce the release of cytokines and inflammatory cells that can increase the ROS in seminal fluid and its toxic effect to sperm (Cho et al. 2016).

Reflux of Metabolites

In addition to previously mentioned hypothesis explaining varicocele impact on fertility, it was reported that incompetent internal spermatic vein allowed the retrograde flow of toxic metabolites from the kidney and adrenal gland. It was reported that catecholamine's reflux damaged spermatogenesis. Another study found that men with varicocele can have an elevated prostaglandin level in spermatic venous blood which can induce ROS that had a deleterious effect on spermatogenesis (Cohen et al. 1985; Ito et al. 1982). On the other hand an experimental study showed no changes of varicocele impact on the testis after left adrenalectomy (Harrison et al. 1986; Sofikitis, N., and I. Miyagawa 1993). Therefore, still the pathophysiology of reflux and the metabolites effect need more investigation.

Apoptosis

Varicocele associated apoptosis and its impact on male fertility has been recognized (Chang et al. 2010). Apoptosis is normal phenomenon. The apoptotic sperm cells in ejaculate tend to be higher in varicocele cases than in fertile control men (Ku et al. 2005). Tissue undergoing apoptosis showed accumulation of toxic materials and heavy metals, therefore several studies evaluated its presence in testicular tissue in varicocele cases (Ku et al. 2005). It has been reported that cadmium and apoptosis were in higher level in men with varicocele than in obstructive azoospermia, and those decreased after varicocele repair (Benoff et al. 2005; Benoff et al. 2004). Also, it was demonstrated that cadmium will reduce zinc concentration and enhance ROS production that can negatively affect spermatogenesis (Benoff et al. 1997).

Reactive Oxygen Species and Oxidative Stress

The association of varicocele with increasing ROS has been reported by many studies (Romeo et al. 2003; Alkan et al. 2018). This relationship has been demonstrated by presence of high level of ROS in infertile men with varicocele than in those without varicocele (Sakamoto et al. 2008). The ROS are oxidizing agents that result from metabolism of oxygen, and at least they have one unpaired electron that makes them reactive species, which will be highly reactive in the presence of amino acids, lipids, and nucleic acids (Sharma and Agarwal 1996). They include superoxide anion (O2-), hydrogen peroxide (H_2O_2), and the hydroxyl radical (OH). There are some other species that contain nitrogen atoms such as NO, nitrate (NO3-), nitroxide (NO-), *nitrous oxide* (N_2O), and nitroxyl (HNO) (Cho et al. 2016; Alkan et al. 2018). Normally in human reproductive system there is a balance between ROS and antioxidant scavenging system which is called oxidative stress status. Although for normal sperm functions like sperm capacitation, acrosome reaction and sperm-oocyte fusion there is an essential need for small physiological level of ROS (Alkan et al. 2018; Sharma and Agarwal 1996), however, excessive production of ROS in semen will cause impaired spermatogenesis, abnormal spermatozoa and increase in leukocytes. This will overwhelm the defense mechanism of antioxidants that will lead to increased oxidative stress (Zini, Lamirande, and Gagnon; 1993; John Aitken, Clarkson, and Fishel 1989; Ochsendorf 1999).

There are several mechanisms for OS to produce negative impact on sperm. The ROS increase the peroxidation of the polyunsaturated fatty acids of the sperm cell membrane that can lead to structural damage of sperm head and mid-piece membrane which will affect its fertilization potential (Griveau et al. 1995). In addition, OS can impair sperm motility by damage to axonemal proteins (De Lamirande, and Gagnon 1992). The OS impacts on DNA are well documented (Sun, Jurisicova, and Casper 1997). The DNA damage can occur both on an amino acid or the backbone that will lead to mature sperm DNA fragmentation and apoptosis (Agarwal, Saleh, and Bedaiwy 2003; Barzilai and Yamamoto 2004). The damage can be obvious in the Yq chromosome where the AZF region is located, which can result in azoospermia in offspring (Agarwal, Hamada, and Esteves 2012). Despite that OS and its effects on spermatozoa are known, the possible mechanism in which varicocele increases OS remains unclear and still under investigation. The OS in semen cannot be measured directly; therefore excess production of ROS or inability of antioxidant volume to buffer it will reflect the increase in OS. There are several tests which measure the ROS either by direct or indirect assay.

SPERM DNA FRAGMENTATION

Sperm DNA integrity is crucial for subsequent fertilization and normal embryonal development, thus the consequences of damaged DNA in male gamete is infertility, miscarriage, offspring birth defect, and diminished fertility in ART (Aitken, De Iuliis, and McLachlan 2009; Esteves et al. 2014). There is a negative correlation between DNA fragmentation and semen quality specially sperm concentration. A high level of DNA fragmentation can be found in one quarter of men in couples with unexplained infertility (IRVINE et al. 2000, Oleszczuk et al. 2013). Although naturally the sperm and oocysts can repair damaged DNA by special enzymes and mechanisms, such mechanisms cannot repair all damaged DNA (Agarwal, Hamada, and Esteves 2012). Several studies have reported the relation between varicocele and sperm DNA fragmentation. It has been demonstrated that fertile and infertile men with varicocele tend to have higher DNA fragmentation than those without varicocele (Zini and Dohle 2011). The germ cell DNA fragmentation can happen in the testis and excurrent ducts. It has been reported that sperm DNA fragmentation is more in epididymis and ejaculated sperm than in the testis (Moskovtsev et al. 2010; Esteves et al. 2015). The generation of sperm DNA fragmentation has been explained by the hypothesis of abortive apoptosis and maturation defects (Sakkas et al. 1999; Sakkas et al. 1995). The ROS impact on DNA has been well reported and they are considered as major element in sperm DNA fragmentation. It is hypothesized that the first step in the DNA damage process is defect in chromatin remodeling which will lead to reduced protamination efficiency before chromatin is attacked by ROS (Aitken and De Iuliis 2009). The ROS damage the DNA by insulting the base and backbone. This damage includes point mutations, polymorphisms, deletions, chromosomal rearrangements, frame shifts and single-stranded or double-stranded breaks (Aitken and Krausz 2001). The measurement of DNA fragmentation can be achieved by flow cytometry, and or fluorescence microscopy utilizing different techniques, such as sperm chromatin structure assay (SCSA), terminal deoxynucleotidyl transferase-mediated fluorescein-dUTP nick-end labeling (TUNEL) assay, (COMET) assay, and sperm chromatin dispersion (SCD) assay (Cho et al. 2016).

DNA Fragmentation Impact on Outcome

The negative impact of Sperm DNA fragmentation on sperm quality and semen parameters has been extensively reported. Beyond that it had been demonstrated that this damage can negatively correlate with embryo quality, blastocyst formation, embryo implantation, and clinical pregnancy rates (Zheng et al. 2018). The increased oxidative DNA damage in sperm shows negative effect on male offspring fertility, and also may cause cancer in offspring (Lewis and Kumar 2015). Experimental study of a long-term effects of mouse intracytoplasmic sperm injection (ICSI) with DNA fragmented sperm demonstrated reduction in embryo development, number of pups, longevity, development of atypical tumors, and altered behavioral responses (Fernández-Gonzalez et al. 2008). On the other hand a systemic review indicates that the available studies are heterogeneous with no consistent relationship between sperm DNA damage and embryo quality and/or development in ART, with the data suggesting that the influence maybe more significant in ICSI than in in vitro fertilization (IVF) (Zini et al. 2011). Although the impact of sperm DNA damage on ART remains controversial, there is sufficient evidence proving this relation. A met-analysis showed that a high level of sperm DNA fragmentation has a detrimental impact on the outcome of ART by decreasing pregnancy rate and increasing the miscarriage rate (Simon et al. 2017; Zhao et al. 2014).

VARICOCELE REPAIR CLINICAL OUTCOME

Consideration of varicocele repair in male partner of a couple attempting to conceive is recommended only if all of the following conditions are present; a palpable varicocele, couple has known infertility, female partner has a normal fertility or potentially treatable cause of infertility, and a male partner with one or more abnormal semen parameters or abnormal result from sperm function test. An adult male presenting with palpable varicocele and abnormal semen analyses is a candidate for varicocele repair even if he has no plan to conceive currently but has a desire for future fertility. In addition, there are few points to be considered in the decision of varicocele repair such as female partner's age, and the period during which the couple has failed to conceive (Cocuzza et al. 2008).

The varicocele repair is a ligation with or without division of clinical varicocele. Several nonsurgical and surgical approaches have been advocated, including varicocele embolization, laparoscopic repair, and surgical ligation with or without microscope in the retroperitoneum, inguinal canal or subinguinally. The best outcomes have been reported after microsurgical techniques (Al Bakri et al. 2012; Diegidio et al. 2011). Although the effect of varicocele repair on semen analysis is controversial, the favorable outcome is mostly reported (Shabana et al. 2015). The improvement of sperm concentration, motility and morphology was significantly demonstrated after surgical varicocele repair (Agarwal et al. 2007). The current evidence confirms reduction in oxidative induced sperm DNA damage after surgical varicocele repair by ameliorating OS markers and consequently the sperm DNA integrity (Roque and Esteves 2018; Vakalopoulos et al.2017). This beneficial effect is also noticed on sperm maturation, improvement of DNA integrity and chromatin compaction (Alhathal, San Gabriel, and Zini 2016). The varicocele repair will significantly improve the semen parameters and decrease DNA fragmentation rate, furthermore it was reported that low DNA fragmentation index values after varicocele repair are associated with increased pregnancy rate, as 37% of couples will have spontaneous pregnancy, and 24% achieved pregnancy with ART (Smit et al. 2010). Randomized controlled trials reported significant increase of natural pregnancy rate after varicocele repair (Cocuzza, Tiseo, and Esteves 2016).

Assisted Reproductive Technology Outcome before and after Varicocele Repair

The treatment options for couples with male infertility associated with varicocele, include varicocele repair, and ART. The ART is performed for couples with infertility that cannot achieve pregnancy naturally. The ART includes several techniques such as IVF embryo transfer (ET), ICSI and ET, and intrauterine insemination (IUI) which is a simplest form of ART. The couple's choice of treatment method can be influenced by several factors. The untreated varicocele can negatively impact semen parameters and future fertility (Cocuzza et al. 2008). The varicocele repair can be a permanent cure for infertility, or can increase the fertility potential. The repair is a considerable choice especially for those couples who plan to have more than one child. The couples who choose ART may need to repeat the process. Also, age of the female partner can be an additional factor (Cocuzza et al. 2008).

The varicocele repair is not usually indicated when ART procedure is planed for treatment of female infertility. It can be considered in certain circumstances. It was demonstrated that the varicocele repair can restore sperm to normal ejaculate in men with non-obstructive azoospermia, which can limit or obviate the need for testicular sperm aspiration or extraction in ART (Matthews, Matthews, and Goldstein 1998; KIM et al. 1999). It has been reported that after varicocele repair 57.6% of men who initially were candidates for IUI, got upgraded to natural pregnancy, and 53.2% of men who were initially candidates for IVF were upgraded to IUI or natural pregnancy (Samplaski et al. 2017). A recent study demonstrated that varicocele repair can increase pregnancy and live birth rate after IUI, even when semen parameters showed no improvement, which suggests that the increase in pregnancy rates may be related to functional factors such DNA integrity and OS that cannot be assessed by basic semen analysis (Table 1, Daitch et al. 2001; Penson et al. 2002; Çayan et al. 2002).

It has been reported that varicocele repair is more cost-effective than primary treatment with ART. Also it was found that varicocele repair in combination with IUI in men with clinical varicocele is more cost-effective than direct IVF or ICSI (Schlegel 1997; Kim 2013; Dubin et al. 2018).

Table 1. ART outcome before and after varicocele repair

Study (n)	***Groups**	****Parameter**	**Result (%)**
Esteves et al., 2010 (n = 242)	A (*n* = 80) vs B (*n*=162)	FR	78 vs 66 (*P* = 0.04)
		IR	
		CPR	60.0 vs 45.1 (*P* = 0.04)
		LBR	46.3 vs 31.5 (*P* = 0.03)
		MR	22.9 vs 30.1 (*P* = 0.46)
Gokce et al., 2013 (n = 306)	A (*n* = 168) vs B (*n* = 138)	FR	
		IR	
		CPR	62.5 vs 47.1 (*P* = 0.001)
		LBR	47.56 vs 29.0 (*P* =0.0002)
		MR	14.9 vs 18.1 (*P* = 0.057)
Shiraishi et al., 2012 (n = 74)	A (*n* = 21) vs B (*n* = 53)	FR	70.3 vs 68.8 (*P* = 0.93)
		IR	
		CPR	61.9 vs 28.3 (*P* = 0.02)
		LBR	52.3 vs 24.5 (*P* = 0.04)
		MR	
Pasqualotto et al., 2012 (n = 248)	A (*n* = 169) vs B (*n* = 79)	FR	64.9 vs 73.2 (*P* = 0.037)
		IR	22.1 vs 17.3 (*P* =0.5882)
		CPR	30.9 vs 31.1 (*P* = 0.98)
		LBR	
		MR	23.9 vs 21.7 (*P* = 0.84)
Daitch et al. 2001 (n = 58)	C (*n* = 34) vs D (*n* = 24)	FR	
		IR	
		CPR	11.8 vs 6.3 (*P* = 0.04)
		LBR	23.9 vs 21.7 (*P* = 0.007)
		MR	

* Groups: A = ICSI with prior varicocele repair, B = ICSI without prior varicocele repair, C = IUI with prior varicocele repair, D = IUI without prior varicocele repair.

** Parameter: FR = Fertilization Rate, IR = Implantation R, CPR = Clinical Pregnancy Rate, LBR = Live Birth Rate, and MR = Miscarriage Rate.

The relation between varicocele, sperm DNA integrity, and ART outcomes occupied researchers concern. As we mentioned earlier in this chapter, OS and elevated sperm DNA fragmentation have been associated with infertility related to varicocele. Although sperm with fragmented DNA and sperm without DNA fragmentation apparently can fertilize oocytes with similar efficiency, it has been demonstrated that high DNA fragmentation negatively impacts embryo development and may jeopardize pregnancy outcomes in ART (Avendaño et al. 2010; Robinson et al. 2012). Therefore, surgical varicocele repair before ART may out perform the direct resorting to ART without varicocele repair.

There are several studies reporting the outcome significance of ICSI with and without prior varicocele repair for men with nonobstructive azoospermia. However, a few studies provide information about the interval between varicocele repair and ICSI. One study recommended this interval to be 6.2 months, while it was 7.2 ± 2.8 months in the other study (Esteves, Oliveira, and Bertolla 2010; Gokce et al. 2013). Microsurgical subinguinal varicocele repair as the surgical approach, also has been included in some of these studies (Esteves, Oliveira, and Bertolla 2010; Gokce et al. 2013; Pasqualotto et al. 2012). These studies showed performing varicocele repair in patients with clinical varicocele prior to ICSI is associated with statistically significant increase in the clinical pregnancy rate, and live birth rates (Esteves, Oliveira, and Bertolla 2010; Gokce et al. 2013; Shiraishi, Matsuyama, and Takihara 2012). Also, it has been found that varicocele repair before ICSI can statistically increase fertilization rate and decrease miscarriage rate (Esteves, Oliveira, and Bertolla 2010). There are other studies which found non significant differences between the two groups for clinical pregnancy, implantation, and miscarriage rates (Pasqualotto et al. 2012; Shiraishi, Matsuyama, and Takihara 2012). A systematic review and metanalysis found a significant improvement in pregnancy outcomes by ICSI if varicocele repair was performed prior to ICSI (Esteves, Roque, and Agarwal 2016).

CONCLUSION

The varicocele is common surgically correctable cause of male infertility. There are several hypotheses explaining the negative impact of varicocele on semen parameters, and sperm function, which can improve significantly after varicocele repair. It was demonstrated that varicocele repair can increase the rate of spontaneous pregnancy, likewise there are evidences showing increase in pregnancy and live birth rate if performed prior to ART. The other studies reported that varicocele repair in conjunction with ART is more cost-effective than attempting treatment with ART without varicocele repair. We should take into consideration that all mentioned factors and outcomes can influence the couple's and treating team's decision when treating infertile couples by ART with abnormal semen parameters or sperm function tests associated with varicocele.

REFERENCES

[1] Agarwal A, Sharma R, Harlev A, Esteves SC. Effect of varicocele on semen characteristics according to the new 2010 World Health Organization criteria: a systematic review and meta-analysis. *Asian journal of andrology*. 2016 Mar;18(2):163.

[2] Agarwal A, Saleh RA, Bedaiwy MA. Role of reactive oxygen species in the pathophysiology of human reproduction. *Fertility and sterility*. 2003 Apr 1;79(4):829-43.

[3] Agarwal A, Hamada A, Esteves SC. Insight into oxidative stress in varicocele-associated male infertility: part 1. *Nature Reviews Urology*. 2012 Dec;9(12):678.

[4] Agarwal A, Deepinder F, Cocuzza M, Agarwal R, Short RA, Sabanegh E, Marmar JL. Efficacy of varicocelectomy in improving semen parameters: new meta-analytical approach. *Urology*. 2007 Sep 1;70(3):532-8.

[5] Aitken RJ, De Iuliis GN, McLachlan RI. Biological and clinical significance of DNA damage in the male germ line. *International journal of andrology*. 2009 Feb;32(1):46-56.

[6] Aitken RJ, De Iuliis GN. On the possible origins of DNA damage in human spermatozoa. *MHR: Basic science of reproductive medicine*. 2009 Jul 31;16(1):3-13.
[7] Aitken RJ, Krausz C. Oxidative stress, DNA damage and the Y chromosome. *REPRODUCTION-CAMBRIDGE-*. 2001 Oct 1;122(4):497-506.
[8] Al Bakri A, Lo K, Grober E, Cassidy D, Cardoso JP, Jarvi K. Time for improvement in semen parameters after varicocelectomy. *The Journal of urology*. 2012 Jan;187(1):227-31.
[9] Alhathal N, San Gabriel M, Zini A. Beneficial effects of microsurgical varicocoelectomy on sperm maturation, DNA fragmentation, and nuclear sulfhydryl groups: a prospective trial. *Andrology*. 2016 Nov;4(6):1204-8.
[10] Alkan İ, Yüksel M, Canat HL, Atalay HA, Can O, Özveri H, Başar MM. Superoxide anion production by the spermatozoa of men with varicocele: relationship with varicocele grade and semen parameters. *The world journal of men's health*. 2018 Sep;36(3): 255.
[11] Avendaño C, Franchi A, Duran H, Oehninger S. DNA fragmentation of normal spermatozoa negatively impacts embryo quality and intracytoplasmic sperm injection outcome. *Fertility and sterility*. 2010 Jul 1;94(2):549-57.
[12] Alsaikhan B, Alrabeeah K, Delouya G, Zini A. Epidemiology of varicocele. *Asian journal of andrology*. 2016 Mar;18(2):179.
[13] Baigorri BF, Dixon RG. *Men's Health: Varicocele: A Review. InSeminars in interventional radiology* 2016 Sep (Vol. 33, No. 3, p. 170). Thieme Medical Publishers.
[14] Barzilai A, Yamamoto KI. DNA damage responses to oxidative stress. *DNA repair*. 2004 Aug 1;3(8-9):1109-15.
[15] Benoff S, Goodwin LO, Millan C, Hurley IR, Pergolizzi RG, Marmar JL. Deletions in L-type calcium channel α1 subunit testicular transcripts correlate with testicular cadmium and apoptosis in infertile men with varicoceles. *Fertility and sterility*. 2005 Mar 1;83(3):622-34.
[16] Benoff SH, Millan C, Hurley IR, Napolitano B, Marmar JL. Bilateral increased apoptosis and bilateral accumulation of cadmium in

infertile men with left varicocele. *Human Reproduction*. 2004 Mar 1;19(3):616-27.

[17] Benoff S, Hurley IR, Barcia M, Mandel FS, Cooper GW, Hershlag A. A potential role for cadmium in the etiology of varicoceleassociated infertility. *Fertility and sterility*. 1997 Feb 1;67(2):336-47.

[18] Braedel HU, Steffens J, Ziegler M, Polsky MS, Platt ML. A possible ontogenic etiology for idiopathic left varicocele. *The Journal of urology*. 1994 Jan 1;151(1):62-6.

[19] Çayan S, Erdemir F, Özbey IS, Turek PJ, Kadioğlu A, Tellaloğlu S. Can varicocelectomy significantly change the way couples use assisted reproductive technologies?. *The Journal of urology*. 2002 Apr 1;167(4):1749-52.

[20] Chang FW, Sun GH, Cheng YY, Chen IC, Chien HH, Wu GJ. Effects of varicocele upon the expression of apoptosis-related proteins. *Andrologia*. 2010 Aug;42(4):225-30.

[21] Cho CL, Esteves SC, Agarwal A. Novel insights into the pathophysiology of varicocele and its association with reactive oxygen species and sperm DNA fragmentation. *Asian Journal of Andrology*. 2016 Mar;18(2):186.

[22] Cocuzza M, Cocuzza MA, Bragais FM, Agarwal A. The role of varicocele repair in the new era of assisted reproductive technology. *Clinics*. 2008;63(3):395-404.

[23] Comhaire F, Vermeulen A. Varicocele sterility: cortisol and catecholamines. *Fertility and sterility*. 1974 Jan 1;25(1):88-95.

[24] Cohen MS, Plaine L, Brown JS. The role of internal spermatic vein plasma catecholamine determinations in subfertile men with varicoceles. *Fertility and sterility*. 1975 Dec 1;26(12):1243-9.

[25] Daitch, J. A., Mohamed A. B, Eleonora B. P, Benjamin N. H., Jorge H., Tommaso F, Anthony J. T, David R. N, Ashok A. "Varicocelectomy improves intrauterine insemination success rates in men with varicocele." *The Journal of urology* 165, no. 5 (2001): 1510-1513.

[26] De Lamirande, E. V. E., Claude G. "Reactive oxygen species and human spermatozoa. II. Depletion of adenosine triphosphate plays an important role in the inhibition of sperm motility." *Journal of andrology* 13, no. 5 (1992): 379-386.

[27] Diegidio P, Jhaveri JK, Ghannam S, Pinkhasov R, Shabsigh R, Fisch H. Review of current varicocelectomy techniques and their outcomes. *BJU international*. 2011 Oct;108(7):1157-72.
[28] Dubin JM, Greer AB, Kohn TP, Masterson TA, Ji L, Ramasamy R. Men with severe oligospermia appear to benefit from varicocele repair: a cost-effectiveness analysis of assisted reproductive technology. *Urology*. 2018 Jan 1;111:99-103.
[29] El-Domyati MM, Al-Din AB, Barakat MT, El-Fakahany HM, Honig S, Xu J, Sakkas D. The expression and distribution of deoxyribonucleic acid repair and apoptosis markers in testicular germ cells of infertile varicocele patients resembles that of old fertile men. *Fertility and sterility*. 2010 Feb 1;93(3):795-801.
[30] Esteves SC, Sharma RK, Gosálvez J, Agarwal A. A translational medicine appraisal of specialized andrology testing in unexplained male infertility. *International urology and nephrology*. 2014 Jun 1;46(6):1037-52.
[31] Esteves SC, Sánchez-Martín F, Sánchez-Martín P, Schneider DT, Gosálvez J. Comparison of reproductive outcome in oligozoospermic men with high sperm DNA fragmentation undergoing intracytoplasmic sperm injection with ejaculated and testicular sperm. *Fertility and sterility*. 2015 Dec 1;104(6):1398-1405.
[32] Esteves SC, Oliveira FV, Bertolla RP. Clinical outcome of intracytoplasmic sperm injection in infertile men with treated and untreated clinical varicocele. *The Journal of urology*. 2010 Oct;184(4):1442-6.
[33] Esteves SC, Roque M, Agarwal A. Outcome of assisted reproductive technology in men with treated and untreated varicocele: systematic review and meta-analysis. *Asian Journal of Andrology*. 2016 Mar;18(2):254.
[34] Fernández-Gonzalez R, Moreira PN, Pérez-Crespo M, Sánchez-Martín M, Ramirez MA, Pericuesta E, Bilbao A, Bermejo-Alvarez P, Hourcade JD, Fonseca FR, Gutiérrez-Adán A. Long-term effects of mouse intracytoplasmic sperm injection with DNA-fragmented sperm on health and behavior of adult offspring. *Biology of reproduction*. 2008 Apr 1;78(4):761-72.

[35] Gat Y, Gornish M, Navon U, Chakraborty J, Bachar GN, Ben-Shlomo I. Right varicocele and hypoxia, crucial factors in male infertility: fluid mechanics analysis of the impaired testicular drainage system. *Reproductive biomedicine online*. 2006 Jan 1;13(4):510-5.

[36] Gokce MI, Gülpınar Ö, Süer E, Mermerkaya M, Aydos K, Yaman Ö. Effect of performing varicocelectomy before intracytoplasmic sperm injection on clinical outcomes in non-azoospermic males. *International urology and nephrology*. 2013 Apr;45(2):367-72.

[37] Griveau JF, Dumont E, Renard P, Callegari JP, Le Lannou D. *Reactive oxygen species, lipid peroxidation and enzymatic defence systems in human spermatozoa.* Reproduction. 1995 Jan 1;103(1):17-26.

[38] Hamada A, Esteves SC, Agarwal A. Insight into oxidative stress in varicocele-associated male infertility: part 2. *Nature* Reviews Urology. 2013 Jan;10(1):26.

[39] Harrison RM, Lewis RW, Roberts JA. Pathophysiology of varicocele in nonhuman primates: long-term seminal and testicular changes. *Fertility and sterility*. 1986 Sep 1;46(3):500-10.

[40] Ikeda M, Kodama H, Fukuda J, Shimizu Y, Murata M, Kumagai J, Tanaka T. Role of radical oxygen species in rat testicular germ cell apoptosis induced by heat stress. *Biology of reproduction*. 1999 Aug 1;61(2):393-9.

[41] Irvine, D. S, Jeremy P. Twigg, E L. Gordon, N F, Philip A. M, and R. J Aitken. "DNA integrity in human spermatozoa: relationships with semen quality." *Journal of andrology* 21, no. 1 (2000): 33-44.

[42] Ito H, Fuse H, Minagawa H, Kawamura K, Murakami M, Shimazaki J. Internal spermatic vein prostaglandins in varicocele patients. *Fertility and sterility*. 1982 Feb 1;37(2):218-22.

[43] John Aitken R, Clarkson JS, Fishel S. Generation of reactive oxygen species, lipid peroxidation, and human sperm function. *Biology of reproduction*. 1989 Jul 1;41(1):183-97.

[44] Khera M, Lipshultz LI. Evolving approach to the varicocele. *Urologic Clinics of North America*. 2008 May 1;35(2):183-9.

[45] Kim KH, Lee JY, Kang DH, Lee H, Seo JT, Cho KS. Impact of surgical varicocele repair on pregnancy rate in subfertile men with clinical varicocele and impaired semen quality: a meta-analysis of

randomized clinical trials. *Korean journal of urology*. 2013 Oct;54(10):703.

[46] Kim JH. Surgical managements versus artificial reproductive technology in male infertility: cost effectiveness in Korea. *Clin Exp Reprod Med*. 2013;40:30-5.

[47] Kim ED, Leibman BB, Grinblat DM, Lipshultz LI. Varicocele repair improves semen parameters in azoospermic men with spermatogenic failure. *The Journal of urology*. 1999 Sep;162(3 Part 1):737-40.

[48] Kirby EW, Wiener LE, Rajanahally S, Crowell K, Coward RM. Undergoing varicocele repair before assisted reproduction improves pregnancy rate and live birth rate in azoospermic and oligospermic men with a varicocele: a systematic review and meta-analysis. *Fertility and sterility*. 2016 Nov 1;106(6):1338-43.

[49] Ku JH, Shim HB, Kim SW, Paick JS. The role of apoptosis in the pathogenesis of varicocele. *BJU international*. 2005 Nov;96(7): 1092-6.

[50] Lee JD, Jeng SY, Lee TH. Increased expression of hypoxia-inducible factor-1α in the internal spermatic vein of patients with varicocele. *The Journal of urology*. 2006 Mar;175(3):1045-8.

[51] Lewis SE, Kumar K. The paternal genome and the health of the assisted reproductive technology child. *Asian journal of andrology*. 2015 Jul;17(4):616.

[52] Lipshultz LI, Howards SS, Niederberger CS, editors. *Infertility in the Male*. Cambridge University Press; 2009 Sep 24.

[53] Marmar JL, Agarwal A, Prabakaran S, Agarwal R, Short RA, Benoff S, Thomas Jr AJ. Reassessing the value of varicocelectomy as a treatment for male subfertility with a new meta-analysis. *Fertility and sterility*. 2007 Sep 1;88(3):639-48.

[54] Matthews GJ, Matthews ED, Goldstein M. Induction of spermatogenesis and achievement of pregnancy after microsurgical varicocelectomy in men with azoospermia and severe oligoasthenospermia. *Fertility and sterility*. 1998 Jul 1;70 (1):71-5.

[55] Mitropoulos D, Deliconstantinos G, Zervas A, Villiotou V, Dimopoulos C, Stavrides J. Nitric oxide synthase and xanthine oxidase activities in the spermatic vein of patients with varicocele:

a potential role for nitric oxide and peroxynitrite in sperm dysfunction. *The Journal of urology*. 1996 Dec;156(6):1952-8.
[56] Miyaoka R, Esteves SC. A critical appraisal on the role of varicocele in male infertility. *Advances in urology*. 2011 Nov 28;2012.
[57] Morgan D, Cherny VV, Murphy R, Xu W, Thomas LL, DeCoursey TE. Temperature dependence of NADPH oxidase in human eosinophils. *The Journal of physiology*. 2003 Jul;550(2):447-58.
[58] Moskovtsev SI, Jarvi K, Mullen JB, Cadesky KI, Hannam T, Lo KC. Testicular spermatozoa have statistically significantly lower DNA damage compared with ejaculated spermatozoa in patients with unsuccessful oral antioxidant treatment. *Fertility and sterility*. 2010 Mar 1;93(4):1142-6.
[59] Ochsendorf FR. Infections in the male genital tract and reactive oxygen species. *Human Reproduction Update*. 1999 Sep 1;5(5):399-420.
[60] Oleszczuk K, Augustinsson L, Bayat N, Giwercman A, Bungum M. Prevalence of high DNA fragmentation index in male partners of unexplained infertile couples. *Andrology*. 2013 May;1(3):357-60.
[61] Pasqualotto FF, Braga DP, Figueira RC, Setti AS, Iaconelli Jr A, Borges Jr E. Varicocelectomy does not impact pregnancy outcomes following intracytoplasmic sperm injection procedures. *Journal of andrology*. 2012 Mar 4;33(2):239-43.
[62] Penson DF, Paltiel AD, Krumholz HM, Palter S. The cost-effectiveness of treatment for varicocele related infertility. *The Journal of urology*. 2002 Dec;168(6):2490-4.
[63] Rajfer J, Turner TT, Rivera F, Howards SS, Sikka SC. Inhibition of testicular testosterone biosynthesis following experimental varicocele in rats. *Biology of Reproduction*. 1987 May 1;36(4): 933-7.
[64] Robinson L, Gallos ID, Conner SJ, Rajkhowa M, Miller D, Lewis S, Kirkman-Brown J, Coomarasamy A. The effect of sperm DNA fragmentation on miscarriage rates: a systematic review and meta-analysis. *Human reproduction. 2012* Oct 1;27(10):2908-17.
[65] Romeo C, Ientile R, Impellizzeri P, Turiaco N, Teletta M, Antonuccio P, Basile M, Gentile C. Preliminary report on nitric

oxide-mediated oxidative damage in adolescent varicocele. *Human Reproduction*. 2003 Jan 1;18(1):26-9.

[66] Rosselli M, Dubey RK, Imthurn B, Macas E, Keller PJ. Andrology: effects of nitric oxide on human spermatozoa: evidence that nitric oxide decreases sperm motility and induces sperm toxicity. *Human Reproduction*. 1995 Jul 1;10(7):1786-90.

[67] Roque M, Esteves SC. Effect of varicocele repair on sperm DNA fragmentation: a review. *International urology and nephrology*. 2018 Apr;50(4):583-603.

[68] Sakamoto Y, Ishikawa T, Kondo Y, Yamaguchi K, Fujisawa M. The assessment of oxidative stress in infertile patients with varicocele. *BJU international*. 2008 Jun;101(12):1547-52.

[69] Sakkas D, Mariethoz E, Manicardi G, Bizzaro D, Bianchi PG, Bianchi U. Origin of DNA damage in ejaculated human spermatozoa. *Reviews of reproduction*. 1999 Jan 1;4:31-7.

[70] Sakkas D, Manicardi G, Grace Bianchi P, Bizzaro D, Bianchi U. Relationship between the presence of endogenous nicks and sperm chromatin packaging in maturing and fertilizing mouse spermatozoa. *Biology of Reproduction*. 1995 May 1;52(5):1149-55.

[71] Samplaski MK, Lo KC, Grober ED, Zini A, Jarvi KA. Varicocelectomy to "upgrade" semen quality to allow couples to use less invasive forms of assisted reproductive technology. *Fertility and sterility*. 2017 Oct 1;108(4):609-12.

[72] Setchell BP. Anatomy, vasculature, innervation, and fluids of the male reproductive tract. *The physiology of reproduction*. 1988.

[73] Schlegel PN. Is assisted reproduction the optimal treatment for varicocele-associated male infertility? A cost-effectiveness analysis. *Urology*. 1997 Jan 1;49(1):83-90.

[74] Shabana W, Teleb M, Dawod T, Elsayed E, Desoky E, Shahin A, Eladl M, Sorour W. Predictors of improvement in semen parameters after varicocelectomy for male subfertility: A prospective study. *Canadian Urological Association Journal*. 2015 Sep;9(9-10):E579.

[75] Shiraishi K, Matsuyama H, Takihara H. Pathophysiology of varicocele in male infertility in the era of assisted reproductive

technology. *International journal of urology*. 2012 Jun;19(6):538-50.

[76] Sharma RK, Agarwal A. Role of reactive oxygen species in male infertility. *Urology*. 1996 Dec 1;48(6):835-50.

[77] Simon L, Zini A, Dyachenko A, Ciampi A, Carrell DT. A systematic review and meta-analysis to determine the effect of sperm DNA damage on in vitro fertilization and intracytoplasmic sperm injection outcome. *Asian journal of andrology*. 2017 Jan;19(1):80.

[78] Smit M, Romijn JC, Wildhagen MF, Veldhoven JL, Weber RF, Dohle GR. Decreased sperm DNA fragmentation after surgical varicocelectomy is associated with increased pregnancy rate. *The Journal of urology*. 2010 Jan;183(1):270-4.

[79] Sofikitis N, Dritsas K, Miyagawa I, Koutselinis A. Anatomical characteristics of the left testicular venous system in man. *Archives of andrology*. 1993 Jan 1;30(2):79-85.

[80] Sofikitis N, Miyagawa I. Effects of surgical repair of experimental left varicocele on testicular temperature, spermatogenesis, sperm maturation, endocrine function, and fertility in rabbits. *Archives of andrology*. 1992 Jan 1;29(2):163-75.

[81] Sofikitis N, Miyagawa I. Left adrenalectomy in varicocelized rats does not inhibit the development of varicocele-related physiologic alterations. *International journal of fertility and menopausal studies*. 1993 Jul 1;38(4):250-5.

[82] Sun JG, Jurisicova A, Casper RF. Detection of deoxyribonucleic acid fragmentation in human sperm: correlation with fertilization in vitro. *Biology of reproduction*. 1997 Mar 1;56(3):602-7.

[83] Tiseo BC, Esteves SC, Cocuzza MS. Summary evidence on the effects of varicocele treatment to improve natural fertility in subfertile men. *Asian journal of andrology*. 2016 Mar;18(2):239.

[84] Vakalopoulos I, Kampantais S, Lymperi S, Grivas N, Ioannidis A, Mykoniatis I, Nikolaou V, Dimitriadis G. Should we expand the indications for varicocele treatment?. *Translational andrology and urology*. 2017 Oct;6(5):931.

[85] Yeşilli Ç, Mungan G, Seçkiner I, Akduman B, Açikgöz Ş, Altan K, Mungan A. Effect of varicocelectomy on sperm creatine kinase, HspA2 chaperone protein (creatine kinase-M type), LDH, LDH-X,

and lipid peroxidation product levels in infertile men with varicocele. *Urology*. 2005 Sep 1;66(3):610-5.

[86] Zhao J, Zhang Q, Wang Y, Li Y. Whether sperm deoxyribonucleic acid fragmentation has an effect on pregnancy and miscarriage after in vitro fertilization/intracytoplasmic sperm injection: a systematic review and meta-analysis. *Fertility and sterility*. 2014 Oct 1;102(4):998-1005.

[87] Zheng WW, Song G, Wang QL, Liu SW, Zhu XL, Deng SM, Zhong A, Tan YM, Tan Y. Sperm DNA damage has a negative effect on early embryonic development following in vitro fertilization. *Asian journal of andrology*. 2018 Jan;20(1):75.

[88] Zini A, De Lamirande E, Gagnon C. Reactive oxygen species in semen of infertile patients: levels of superoxide dismutase-and catalase-like activities in seminal plasma and spermatozoa. *International journal of andrology*. 1993 Jun;16(3):183-8.

[89] Zini A, Dohle G. Are varicoceles associated with increased deoxyribonucleic acid fragmentation?. *Fertility and sterility*. 2011 Dec 1;96(6):1283-7.

[90] Zini A, Jamal W, Cowan L, Al-Hathal N. Is sperm DNA damage associated with IVF embryo quality? A systematic review. *Journal of assisted reproduction and genetics*. 2011 May;28(5):391-7.

In: Intracytoplasmic Sperm Injection (ICSI) ISBN: 978-1-53619-762-4
Editor: Murid Javed

Chapter 7

Potential Health Effects of Intracytoplasmic Sperm Injection (ICSI)

Murid Javed**, PhD
Originelle Fertility Clinic and Women's Health Centre,
Ottawa, Canada

Abstract

This chapter highlights the ICSI technique, conventional oocyte fertilization and potential health effects of ICSI. The information is extracted from the published literature and is presented in a way that can be useful not only for the scientists but also for the general reader. Some additional techniques are introduced which are enhancing the usefulness of ICSI. The chapter covers nature of ICSI effects, congenital anomalies, and other major factors that may cause an abnormality in a conceptus. The birth of a healthy child is desire of every parent. In presence of any genetic defect in a parent, the use of sperm selection techniques for ICSI, preimplantation genetic testing and noninvasive prenatal testing are likely to ensure birth of a healthy child.

---

* Corresponding Author's E-mail: murid.javed@gmail.com.

Keywords: congenital abnormality, ICSI, preimplantation genetic testing, birth defects, conceptus, health effects, pregnancy, Y chromosome microdeletions, ICSI children

INTRODUCTION

Intracytoplasmic sperm injection was first used for human oocytes injection in 1992 (Palermo et el, 1992). It was initially intended for semen samples with very low sperm concentration and motility which were not suitable for conventional egg insemination. However, its use has increased exponentially with many in vitro fertilization laboratories exclusively using ICSI. The use of ICSI in the United States of America increased from 36.4% in 1996 to 76.2% in 2012 with the largest increase for cycles without male factor infertility (Boulet et al., 2015) . Although ICSI is an invasive procedure and may cause oocyte damage, it is preferred over the conventional oocyte insemination due to following reasons. It provides more information on the maturity of oocytes. Soon after egg collection, the granulosa cells covering the oocytes are removed and oocytes are evaluated for maturity and presence of any abnormality. The immature oocytes are cultured overnight and injected if attain maturity. For ICSI, only one sperm is needed for each oocyte thus it can be performed in extremely severe male factor infertility cases even with immotile sperm. Surgically retrieved testicular sperm can only be used by ICSI. It avoids polyspermy as in conventional egg insemination more than one sperm can enter the oocyte. The total failed fertilization incidence is only 1-3% after ICSI as compared to 16% after conventional egg insemination (Esfandiari et al., 2005; Barlow et al., 1990).

The ICSI results in higher fertilization (Komsky et al., 2013). Many embryologists remain under stress after performing conventional insemination as the fertilization outcome is unpredictable whereas after performing ICSI, they gain confidence that fertilization will happen. The superiority of ICSI over conventional oocyte insemination for good semen samples is still debatable as ICSI does not increase live birth rate in such cases (Abbas et al., 2020; Boulet et al., 2015; Komsky et al., 2013).

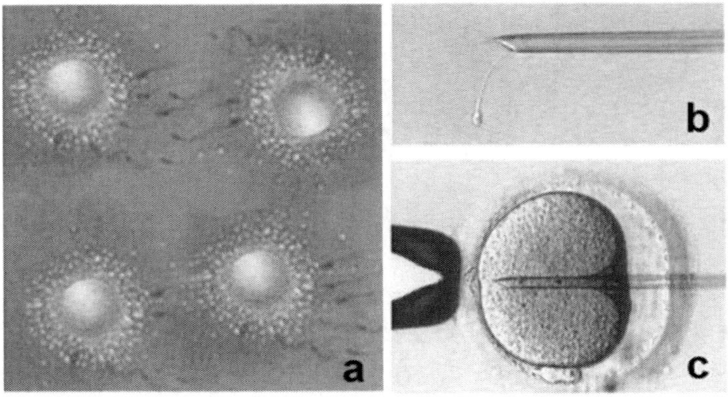

Figure 1. (a) Conventional oocyte insemination. Thousands of sperm are added to the culture medium containing oocytes. The sperm penetrates through cells surrounding oocyte and goes through zona pellucida and egg membrane to cause fertilization. (b) A single sperm is picked into an injection pipette. (c) The injection pipette penetrated through the zona pellucida and egg membrane to deposit the sperm into oocyte cytoplasm.

In the conventional oocyte insemination, the sperm selection is a natural process. The oocytes are incubated with many thousands of sperm allowing natural penetration of sperm through the zona pellucida and the oocyte membrane to result in fertilization (Figure 1a). However in the ICSI (Figure 1b and c), an embryologist selects the sperm and injects into the egg by an injection pipette. In severe male factor cases, a sperm is injected which is unable to cause fertilization by conventional oocyte insemination due to lack of motility, low number or abnormal morphology. Although, at the time of injection, a sperm is magnified usually at 400 X, and is selected based on its motility and morphology, however, the concerns of its ill effects on the health of offspring remain. Also, the severe male factor infertility can be due to genetic defects transmissible to the offspring. The purpose of this chapter is to provide a broader view whether ICSI is causing any ill effects on the health of ICSI conceived children. The information is based on literature review and is summarized into subgroups for a comprehensive overview of the subject.

Nature of ICSI Effects

There are three factors associated with ICSI that may influence the risk of malformation: chromosomal abnormalities in the oocytes and sperm used; drugs used for ovarian stimulation; and the direct injection of sperm into the oocyte (Lacamara et al., 2017). A comprehensive review published by these authors indicated that the combined odds ratio of all studies developed to assess the risk of congenital malformations in ICSI-born infants versus the risk in naturally conceived infants is 1.99 (95% CI [1.87-2.11]) for congenital malformations in ICSI-conceived children when compared to naturally conceived children, which translates into a risk of 7.1% of having a malformation for individuals born after ICSI versus 4.0% for naturally conceived children. The authors cautioned evaluating this result, as comparing data from different studies often brings important methodological implications and difficulties.

Jwa et al., (2019) attempted to distinguish between the effects of treatment (i.e., IVF/ICSI) and that of underlying male subfertility on the risk of major birth defects. The severe oligozoospermia (sperm < 5 × 106/mL) was associated with a significantly increased risk of hypospadias compared with normal sperm concentrations. The ICSI was not associated with any specific major birth defects compared with IVF among cycles with normal sperm concentrations and motility suggesting that underlying male subfertility might affect the risk of major birth defects in relation to ICSI. Further, other factors such as underlying maternal factors, may affect the incidence of this anomaly in babies born following ICSI. The neonatal outcome from the use of testicular sperm from non obstructive azoospermia did not increase birth defects. ICSI with ejaculated spermatozoa from men with Klinefelter's syndrome has low risk of transmission of chromosomal aneuploidy (Yu et al., 2018).

Congenital Abnormalities and Fertilization Method

The congenital anomalies are structural or functional anomalies that occur during intrauterine life and can be identified prenatally, at birth, or later in infancy. Their origin may be genetic or multifactorial, but in most cases the cause is unknown. The concern on safety of ICSI technique has been since its initial use. A number of studies and reviews have been published comparing congenital defects among natural conception, in vitro oocyte insemination and ICSI. Over the past 40 years access of assisted reproduction has increased, and more than 8 million children have been conceived after assisted reproduction technology globally (Wennerholm and Bergh, 2020). The children conceived through assisted reproduction are at increased risk of birth defects as the in vivo conception has failed and sometimes compromised oocytes and sperm are used to create an in vitro embryo. Previously many problems arose as a result of multiple pregnancies as two or more embryos were transferred to achieve higher pregnancy rate. Many countries are now implementing policies for transferring single embryo in <35 years old women. Wennerholm and Bergh (2020) reviewed perinatal outcomes in singletons born after oocyte insemination and ICSI. The pooled estimate for ICSI singletons versus IVF singletons showed a lower risk of preterm birth in ICSI singletons.

The data comparing congenital birth defects after natural or assisted conception is conflicting probably due to the inherent variation in the source and quality of eggs and sperm. Some studies have found no difference for congenital defects between oocyte insemination and ICSI (Han et al., 2018; Zádori et al., 2003; Al-Fifi et al., 2009) whereas other studies found increased birth defects in children conceived by ICSI (Wennerholm and Bergh, 2020; Liberman et al., 2017, Hoorsan et al. 2017, Rimm et al., 2004). The birth-defects usually observed are in central nervous system, eye, ear, face, neck, heart, gastrointestinal system, urinary system, and the musculo-skeletal system, with congenital heart defects being the most common defects. The women seeking assisted reproduction are likely to have an abnormal pregnancy history and are at a higher risk for poor pregnancy conditions and developing pregnancy complications compared to women conceiving spontaneously (Yang et al., 2018).

Y-Chromosome Microdeletions and ICSI Outcome

The AZF region of the Y chromosome is involved in spermatogenesis. Any defect in this region can disturb sperm production. Most Y chromosome microdeletions occur on the long arm of the Y chromosome (Yq11) and are subdivided into 3 AZF regions: a, b, and c (Xi et al., 2019). The defects in AZF region can lead to a higher risk of neuropsychiatry disorders in men. The copy number variations and altered expression of AZF genes are found in several cancers (Colaco and Modi, 2019). The ICSI has enabled men suffering from Y-chromosome microdeletions to have their children, therefore increasing the possibility of these defects to next generation. Several studies have addressed this concern. Some studies have reported similar neonatal and perinatal outcomes after using sperm from patients with or without Y chromosome AZFc microdeletions (Xi et al., 2019, Liu et al., 2013). The challenge in men with Y chromosome AZFc microdeletions is availability of sperm. The ICSI requires only one sperm for each egg and embryologists usually select those with normal morphology and good motility, however, the fear of Y chromosome AZFc microdeletions to offspring remains (Liu et al., 2013). Preimplantation genetic testing (PGT) to identify embryos carrying Y chrosome microdelections is recommended as the Y-chromosome AZFc microdeletions transmitted an abnormal karyotype (inv (9) (p11q13)) to a baby girl, who was conceived after ICSI (Hu et al., 2019).

Imprinting Disorders and ICSI

The genomic imprinting is methylation of cytosine bases in the CpG dinucleotides of DNA which are key regulatory elements of genes. A common process for controlling the gene activity is methylation. A gene that is methylated (inactivated) can be reactivated in male or female gametogenesis for the next generation. Imprinted genes may contribute to behavior and language development, alcohol dependency, schizophrenia, bipolar disorders or to a wide range of malignancies (Butler, 2009). Some studies suggested that ovarian stimulation, culture media used for gametes and early embryos, IVF and ICSI manipulations, and the freezing and thawing of embryos may cause imprinting disorders (Hattori et al., 2019). Tang et al. (2017) suggested that increased imprinting errors in the sperm of infertile patients do not have an obvious influence on ART outcomes or the imprinting of offspring. In this study, the sample size was small as only thirteen samples of cord blood were collected from infants born after ICSI-ET using sperm from infertile men. To establish a reference threshold for the normal methylation status, 30 cord blood samples were collected as controls from naturally conceived healthy newborns. They found that the aberrant methylation of H19 was associated with oligozoospermia and the outcomes did not show significant differences among the IVF-ET control, normal imprinted sperm and abnormal imprinted sperm groups. This study concluded that the effect of paternal sperm imprinting on the imprinting of offspring is limited, although the possibility of direct transmission of imprinting errors is not excluded. It is likely that the imprinting errors in sperm are selectively discarded or corrected during development. Another study reported that the epigenomes of ART and spontaneously conceived children are very similar (El Hajj et al., 2017).

Sperm DNA Fragmentation and ICSI Outcome

DNA fragmentation is accumulation of single- and double-strand DNA breaks. It is a common property of sperm and every man has some degree of sperm DNA fragmentation. The threshold varies depending on what technique is used for determination of sperm DNA fragmentation. One of very commonly used classification is; <15%, 15-30% and >30% DNA fragmentation, referring to good fertility potential, moderate infertility and severe infertility, respectively (Chen et al., 2020). The men with 27–30% DNA fragmentation determined by sperm chromatin structure assay either take longer time to achieve in vivo, intra uterine insemination (IUI) or egg insemination pregnancy or achieve no pregnancy. In such cases ICSI is recommended (Evenson and Wixon 2006; Simon et al., 2019).

For ICSI, usually one sperm is picked based on its motility and morphology under high magnification (usually >200 X). Efforts have been made to determine the DNA integrity of the sperm before injection. A device "PICSI" – physiological intracytoplasmic sperm injection (Figure 2) based on sperm selection by the use of hyaluronan, claims selection of sperm without DNA fragmentation (Miller et al., 2019; Lohinova et al., 2017). Another technique magnetic activated cell sorting (MACS) – which selects non-apoptotic sperm population using Annexin V magnetic beads, has been reported to be equally effective as PICSI (Hasanen et al., 2020).

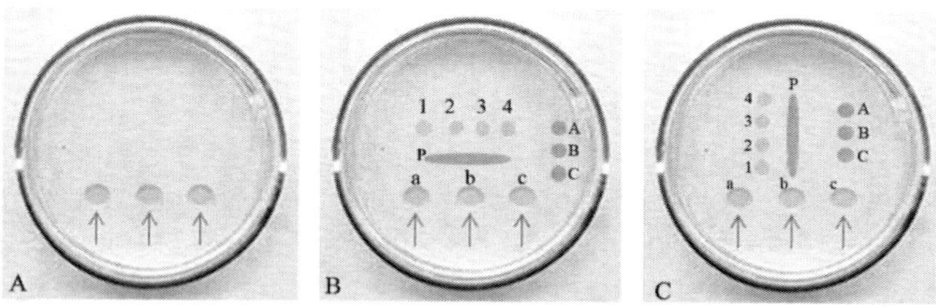

Figure 2. A diagrammatic presentation of a PICSI dish. (A) The 3 arrows point to 3 microdrops of hyaluronan. (B and C) show 2 options of ICSI dish preparation for ICSI. The a, b and c represent hyaluronan drops; P represents PVP drop for immobilizing sperm before ICSI; A,B, C represents drops for washing oocyts and 1,2,3 and 4 are drops to place eggs for ICSI.

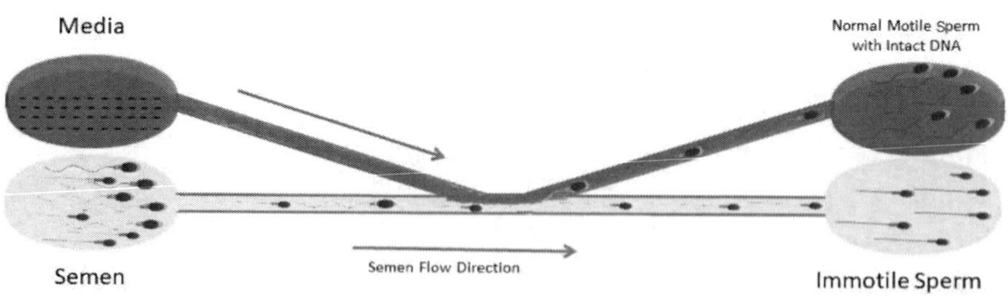

Figure 3. A diagrammatic presentation of a simple microfluidic device. The motile sperm swim up in the media whereas the immotile keep floating straight. This process avoids centrifugation.

Microfluidics (Figure 3), a micro-device known as lab-on-a-chip, selects sperm with intact DNA (Marzano et al., 2020; Bastuba et al., 2020). Higher clinical pregnancy rate, lower miscarriages and higher birth rates have been reported by ICSI using testicular sperm as compared to the ejaculated sperm with high DNA fragmentation (Pabuçcu et al., 2017, Arafa et al., 2018). The sperm retrieved from epididymis and testes can only be used by ICSI.

EDUCATIONAL PERFORMANCE OF ICSI CONCEIVED CHILDREN

Norrman et al., (2020) studied school performance of ICSI conceived children in Sweden. This study included 6,953 singletons born after ICSI, 11, 713 after egg insemination and 2,022,995 after natural conception. The study period was from 1985 to 2006. The study parameters were school performance, parental education, other parental characteristics, child's sex and birth year, maternal smoking during pregnancy, parental age, parity, parental region of birth, parental level of education and frozen embryo transfer. The study indicated that children born after ICSI have similar school performance compared to children born after egg insemination; however, ICSI children had a significantly higher proportion of children qualifying for secondary school and a significantly lower proportion of children with poor school performance than children born after natural conception. One of the limitations of this study is that the infertility diagnoses and indication for ICSI were not available to the authors.

The genetic influence of parental cognitive ability at 5 years age of the child is more important than the mode of conception in determining the long-term intellectual ability of children conceived using ICSI (Leslie et al., 2003). The study of children from 5 European countries (Belgium, Denmark, Greece, Sweden, and the United Kingdom) revealed that motor and cognitive development of ICSI conceived children is very similar to that of naturally conceived children. However, demographic factors such as maternal educational level and maternal age at the time of the birth might play different roles in the cognitive development of ICSI and IVF children, compared with naturally conceived children (Ponjaert-Kristoffersen et al., 2005). Similar results were obtained in other studies (Leunens et al., 2006; Leunens et al., 2008; Place et al., 2003; Steel et al., 2009). The long-term outcome of children born after assisted reproductive technologies regarding neurodevelopment, growth, cardiovascular function, diabetes type 1, asthma, malignancies, and reproductive health, when restricted to singletons, is similar to that of their spontaneously conceived peers (Bergh et al., 2020), however, continuous surveillance of children born after ICSI is needed.

Other Causes of Birth Defects

The birth defects risks could be modifiable or non-modifiable. The modifiable risks may be corrected by thorough patient education and counseling. The risks like age, family history or previously affected child are usually non-modifiable. A strong link has been reported between congenital anomalies and alcohol use, folic acid deficiency, obesity, uncontrolled maternal diabetes mellitus, uncontrolled maternal phenylketonuria, and monozygotic twins. The medicines like angiotensin converting enzyme inhibitors, retinoic acid, folic acid antagonists, and certain anticonvulsants, are also associated with various birth defects (Harris et al., 2017). The folic acid deficiency is reported to cause neural tube and congenital heart defects which can be prevented by folic acid supplementation during early pregnancy (Czeizel et al., 2013).

Maternal or Paternal Age

Due to the wide spread use of ART, the number of older mothers is increasing. The probability of birth defects increases with increased maternal age, male factors and diminished ovarian reserve (Han et al., 2018). The prevalence of chromosomal abnormalities in ART children per pregnancy and per live birth was significantly higher in mothers in the age groups of 30–35 and 40+ years as compared to those <30 yrs

(Ooki, 2013). A study suggested that in cryptozoospermia samples the ICSI with ejaculated sperm should be performed in men < 35 yr old and thereafter testicular sperm should be used as this offers high-quality embryos and higher clinical pregnancy rates (Yu et al., 2019). The Norwegian data on siblings where one child was from ART and the other from spontaneous conception, suggested that low birth weight had a strong link to both maternal and paternal factors (ESHRE Capri Workshop Group, 2014).

Endometriosis

Endometriosis is a condition in which endometrial tissue is present outside the uterine cavity. In a study of 1,495 infants born from women with advanced endometriosis and 27,105 infants born from endometriosis-free women found a 1.557-fold risk that the infants with advanced maternal endometriosis would develop a congenital malformation (Liang et al. 2019). The pelvic endometriosis may interfere with deep placentation and increase risk of obstetrical complications, including preterm birth and antepartum hemorrhage (Brosens et al., 2012). A recent systematic review and meta-analysis reported that endometriosis is associated with an increased risk of gestational hypertension, pre-eclampsia, preterm birth, placenta previa, placental abruption, cesarean section, and stillbirth (Breintoft et al., 2021).

Diabetes

Maternal diabetes has been linked to pregnancy complications and impaired fetal development including growth delay, miscarriage, stillbirth, macrosomia, and congenital malformations. These defects could be due to the effects of diabetes on oogenesis or the pregnancy environment. Tsai et al., (2020) conducted a study on mice to investigate the cause. They artificially induced diabetes in female mice and thereafter used them as oocyte donor or embryo recipient. The embryos were transferred into diabetic and non-diabetic recipients. The diabetic mice oocyte recipients resulted in smaller size fetuses compared to the non-diabetic recipients regardless of the diabetic status of the oocyte donor. Also, the congenital abnormalities were only observed in fetuses carried by the diabetic recipients. The authors concluded that the diabetic status during pregnancy results in restricted fetal growth and congenital deformities.

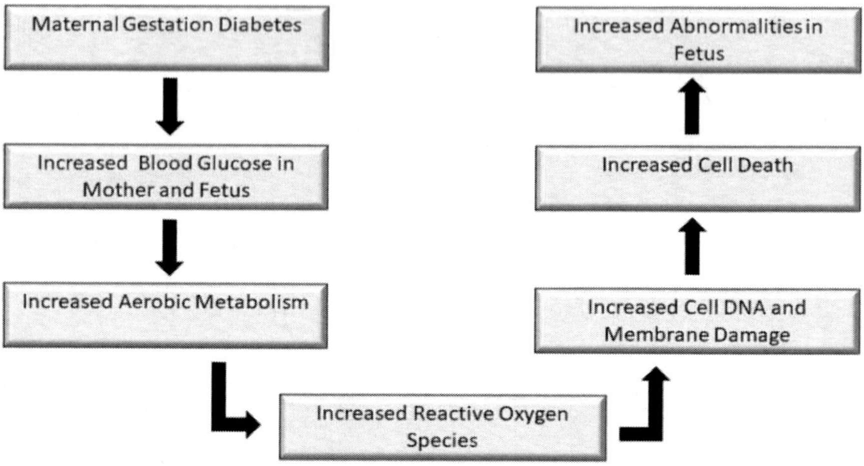

Figure 4. The maternal gestational diabetes increases blood glucose in the mother and fetus which causes increased anaerobic metabolism leading to increased reactive oxygen species which result in increased cell DNA and membrane damage causing cell death that induces increased fetal abnormalities.

In human, diabetes exposes the pregnant mother and the developing fetus to serious health concerns. It may lead to morphological and structural changes in the fetus, leading to abnormal cell death and malformations (Ornoy et al., 2015). The genetic and environmental factors play a critical role in the embryonic and fetal development. The epigenetic changes are inheritable modifications in gene function without a change in nucleotide sequence. Both human and mice studies demonstrated that the maternal environment during gestation can alter the epigenomic landscape and yield long-term phenotypic consequences for the offspring and exposure to hyperglycemia may modify embryonic chromatin. To understand the details of mechanisms involved, the reader is encouraged to consult a comprehensive review by Ornoy et al., 2015. Briefly, the increased blood glucose in the maternal diabetes results in aerobic metabolism that generates increased reactive oxygen species which causes DNA and membrane damage, thus resulting in cell death and fetal defects (Figure 4).

CONCLUSION

The intracytoplasmic sperm injection has proven its usefulness over the past 3 decades. There is still no other technique to replace it. Countless men and infertile women will not be able to parent any child without it. There may be a little increase in congenital abnormalities in children born through ICSI but this could be due to inherent deficiencies in the sperm or egg. More technologies are becoming available to either detect genetic defects in sperm and egg or aid in selection of normal gamete. No study has attributed any congenital abnormality solely because of ICSI technique. The alternate technique, standard IVF or oocyte insemination, has many serious deficiencies and problems due to which the popularity of ICSI is increasing world wide. Utilization of preimplantation genetic testing has further increased use of ICSI as any aneuploid or genetically abnormal embryo can be detected before transfer. Non-invasive prenatal testing is another useful technique to diagnose fetal abnormality as early as 10 weeks of gestation.

REFERENCES

[1] Abbas AM, Hussein RS, Elsenity MA, Samaha II, El Etriby KA, Abd El-Ghany MF, Khalifa MA, Abdelrheem SS, Ahmed AA, Khodry MM. Higher clinical pregnancy rate with in-vitro fertilization versus intracytoplasmic sperm injection in treatment of non-male factor infertility: systematic review and meta-analysis. *Journal of gynecology obstetrics and human reproduction.* 2020 Jun 1;49(6):101706.

[2] Al-Fifi S, Al-Binali A, Al-Shahrani M, Shafiq H, Bahar M, Almushait M, Sobandi L, Eskandar M. Congenital anomalies and other perinatal outcomes in ICSI vs. naturally conceived pregnancies: a comparative study. *Journal of assisted reproduction and genetics*. 2009 Jul;26(7):377-81.

[3] Arafa, M, AlMalki, A, AlBadr, M, Burjaq, H, Majzoub, A, AlSaid, S and Elbardisi, H, 2018. ICSI outcome in patients with high DNA fragmentation: Testicular versus ejaculated spermatozoa. *Andrologia*, *50*(1), p. e12835.

[4] Barlow P, Englert Y, Puissant F, Lejeune B, Delvigne A, Van Rysselberge M, Leroy F. Fertilization failure in IVF: why and what next?. *Human Reproduction*. 1990 May 1;5(4):451-6.

[5] Bastuba, M., Cohen, M., Bastuba, A. and Campbell, P., 2020. Microfluidic sperm separation device dramatically lowers DFI. *Fertility and Sterility*, *113*(4), p. e44.

[6] Bergh C, Wennerholm UB. Long-term health of children conceived after assisted reproductive technology. *Upsala journal of medical sciences*. 2020 Apr 2;125(2):152-7.

[7] Boulet SL, Mehta A, Kissin DM, Warner L, Kawwass JF, Jamieson DJ. Trends in use of and reproductive outcomes associated with intracytoplasmic sperm injection. *Jama*. 2015 Jan 20;313(3):255-63.

[8] Breintoft K, Pinnerup R, Henriksen TB, Rytter D, Uldbjerg N, Forman A, Arendt LH. Endometriosis and Risk of Adverse Pregnancy Outcome: A Systematic Review and Meta-Analysis. *Journal of Clinical Medicine*. 2021 Jan;10(4):667.

[9] Brosens I, Brosens JJ, Fusi L, Al-Sabbagh M, Kuroda K, Benagiano G. Risks of adverse pregnancy outcome in endometriosis. *Fertility and sterility*. 2012 Jul 1;98(1):30-5.

[10] Butler, MG, 2009. Genomic imprinting disorders in humans: a mini-review. *Journal of assisted reproduction and genetics*, *26*(9-10), pp. 477-486.

[11] Chen, L, Fang, J, Jiang, W, Wang, J and Li, D, 2020. Effects of the sperm DNA fragmentation index on the clinical and neonatal outcomes of intracytoplasmic sperm injection cycles. *Journal of Ovarian Research*, *13*, pp. 1-7.

[12] Colaco, S. and Modi, D., 2019. Consequences of Y chromosome microdeletions beyond male infertility. *Journal of Assisted Reproduction and Genetics*, pp. 1-9.

[13] Czeizel AE, Dudás I, Vereczkey A, Bánhidy F. Folate deficiency and folic acid supplementation: the prevention of neural-tube defects and congenital heart defects. *Nutrients.* 2013 Nov;5(11):4760-75.

[14] El Hajj N, Haertle L, Dittrich M, Denk S, Lehnen H, Hahn T, Schorsch M, Haaf T. DNA methylation signatures in cord blood of ICSI children. *Human Reproduction.* 2017 Aug 1;32(8):1761-9.

[15] Esfandiari N, Javed M, Gotlieb L, Casper R. Complete failed fertilization after intracytoplasmic sperm injection-analysis of 10 years' data. International *Journal of Fertility and Womens Medicine.* 2005 Jul 1;50(4):187.

[16] ESHRE Capri Workshop Group piergiorgio. crosignani@ unimi. it. Birth defects and congenital health risks in children conceived through assisted reproduction technology (ART): a meeting report. *Journal of assisted reproduction and genetics.* 2014 Aug;31:947-58.

[17] Evenson, DP and Wixon, R, 2006. Clinical aspects of sperm DNA fragmentation detection and male infertility. *Theriogenology*, *65*(5), pp. 979-991.

[18] Han Y, Luo H, Zhang Y. Congenital anomalies in infants conceived by infertile women through assisted reproductive technology: A cohort study 2004-2014. *Experimental and therapeutic medicine.* 2018 Oct 1;16(4):3179-85.

[19] Harris BS, Bishop KC, Kemeny HR, Walker JS, Rhee E, Kuller JA. Risk factors for birth defects. *Obstetrical & gynecological survey.* 2017 Feb 1;72(2):123-35.

[20] Hasanen, E., Elqusi, K., ElTanbouly, S., AlKhadr, H., Zaki, H., Henkel, R. and Agarwal, A., 2020. PICSI vs. MACS for abnormal sperm DNA fragmentation ICSI cases: a prospective randomized trial. *Journal of Assisted Reproduction and Genetics*, *37*(10), pp. 2605-2613.

[21] Hattori H, Hiura H, Kitamura A, Miyauchi N, Kobayashi N, Takahashi S, Okae H, Kyono K, Kagami M, Ogata T, Arima T.

Association of four imprinting disorders and ART. *Clinical epigenetics.* 2019 Dec;11(1):1-2.

[22] Hoorsan H, Mirmiran P, Chaichian S, Moradi Y, Hoorsan R, Jesmi F. Congenital malformations in infants of mothers undergoing assisted reproductive technologies: A systematic review and meta-analysis study. *Journal of Preventive Medicine and Public Health*. 2017 Nov;50(6):347.

[23] Hu, C, Liu, X, Li, L, Hu, X, Zhu, H, Geng, D, Liu, R and Wang, R, 2019. The reproductive outcome of an infertile man with AZFc microdeletions, via intracytoplasmic sperm injection in a high-risk pregnancy: Case report and literature review. *Medicine*, *98*(28).

[24] Jwa SC, Jwa J, Kuwahara A, Irahara M, Ishihara O, Saito H. Male subfertility and the risk of major birth defects in children born after in vitro fertilization and intracytoplasmic sperm injection: a retrospective cohort study. *BMC pregnancy and childbirth.* 2019 Dec;19(1):1-0.

[25] Komsky-Elbaz A, Raziel A, Friedler S, Strassburger D, Kasterstein E, Komarovsky D, Ron-El R, Ben-Ami I. Conventional IVF versus ICSI in sibling oocytes from couples with endometriosis and normozoospermic semen. *Journal of assisted reproduction and genetics.* 2013 Feb;30(2):251-7.

[26] Lacamara C, Ortega C, Villa S, Pommer R, Schwarze JE. Are children born from singleton pregnancies conceived by ICSI at increased risk for congenital malformations when compared to children conceived naturally? A systematic review and meta-analysis. *JBRA assisted reproduction.* 2017 Jul;21(3):251.

[27] Leslie GI, Gibson FL, McMahon C, Cohen J, Saunders DM, Tennant C. Children conceived using ICSI do not have an increased risk of delayed mental development at 5 years of age. *Human Reproduction.* 2003 Oct 1;18(10):2067-72.

[28] Leunens L, Celestin-Westreich S, Bonduelle M, Liebaers I, Ponjaert-Kristoffersen I. Follow-up of cognitive and motor development of 10-year-old singleton children born after ICSI compared with spontaneously conceived children. *Human Reproduction.* 2008 Jan 1;23(1):105-11.

[29] Leunens L, Celestin-Westreich S, Bonduelle M, Liebaers I, Ponjaert-Kristoffersen I. Cognitive and motor development of 8-

year-old children born after ICSI compared to spontaneously conceived children. *Human Reproduction.* 2006 Nov 1;21(11):2922-9.
[30] Liang Z, Yin M, Ma M, Wang Y, Kuang Y. Effect of Maternal Advanced Endometriosis on Risk of Congenital Malformations for Infants Born After in vitro Fertilization and Frozen–Thawed Embryo Transfer: Analysis of 28,600 Newborns. *Frontiers in endocrinology.* 2019 Nov 12;10:763.
[31] Liberman RF, Getz KD, Heinke D, Luke B, Stern JE, Declercq ER, Chen X, Lin AE, Anderka M. Assisted reproductive technology and birth defects: effects of subfertility and multiple births. *Birth defects research.* 2017 Aug 15;109(14):1144-53.
[32] Liu, XH, Qiao, J, Li, R, Yan, LY and Chen, LX, 2013. Y chromosome AZFc microdeletion may not affect the outcomes of ICSI for infertile males with fresh ejaculated sperm. *Journal of assisted reproduction and genetics*, *30*(6), pp. 813-819.
[33] Lohinova, O., Pitko, V., Sinilo, N., Cherkashyna, Y. and Hanzha, N., 2017. Comparative analysis of sperm selection methods before the intra cytoplasmic sperm injection procedure. *Georgian medical news*, (271), pp. 7-11.
[34] Marzano, G, Chiriacò, MS, Primiceri, E, Dell'Aquila, ME, Ramalho-Santos, J., Zara, V., Ferramosca, A. and Maruccio, G., 2020. Sperm selection in assisted reproduction: A review of established methods and cutting-edge possibilities. *Biotechnology Advances*, *40*, p. 107498.
[35] Miller, D., Pavitt, S., Sharma, V., Forbes, G., Hooper, R., Bhattacharya, S., Kirkman-Brown, J., Coomarasamy, A., Lewis, S., Cutting, R. and Brison, D., 2019. Physiological, hyaluronan-selected intracytoplasmic sperm injection for infertility treatment (HABSelect): a parallel, two-group, randomised trial. *The Lancet*, *393*(10170), pp. 416-422.
[36] Norrman E, Petzold M, Bergh C, Wennerholm UB. School performance in children born after ICSI. *Human Reproduction.* 2020 Feb 29;35(2):340-54.
[37] Ooki S. Maternal age and birth defects after the use of assisted reproductive technology in Japan, 2004–2010. *International journal of women's health.* 2013;5:65.

[38] Ornoy, A, Reece, EA, Pavlinkova, G, Kappen, C, & Miller, RK (2015). Effect of maternal diabetes on the embryo, fetus, and children: congenital anomalies, genetic and epigenetic changes and developmental outcomes. *Birth Defects Research Part C: Embryo Today: Reviews*, *105*(1), 53-72.

[39] Pabuçcu, EG, Caglar, GS, Tangal, S., Haliloglu, AH and Pabuçcu, R., 2017. Testicular versus ejaculated spermatozoa in ICSI cycles of normozoospermic men with high sperm DNA fragmentation and previous ART failures. *Andrologia*, *49*(2), p. e12609.

[40] Palermo G, Joris H, Devroey P, Van Steirteghem AC. Pregnancies after intracytoplasmic injection of single spermatozoon into an oocyte. *The Lancet*. 1992 Jul 4;340 (8810): 17-8.

[41] Place I, Englert Y. A prospective longitudinal study of the physical, psychomotor, and intellectual development of singleton children up to 5 years who were conceived by intracytoplasmic sperm injection compared with children conceived spontaneously and by in vitro fertilization. *Fertility and sterility*. 2003 Dec 1;80(6):1388-97.

[42] Ponjaert-Kristoffersen I, Bonduelle M, Barnes J, Nekkebroeck J, Loft A, Wennerholm UB, Tarlatzis BC, Peters C, Hagberg BS, Berner A, Sutcliffe AG. International collaborative study of intracytoplasmic sperm injection–conceived, in vitro fertilization–conceived, and naturally conceived 5-year-old child outcomes: Cognitive and motor assessments. *Pediatrics*. 2005 Mar 1;115(3):e283-9.

[43] Rimm AA, Katayama AC, Diaz M, Katayama KP. A meta-analysis of controlled studies comparing major malformation rates in IVF and ICSI infants with naturally conceived children. *Journal of assisted reproduction and genetics*. 2004 Dec;21(12):437-43.

[44] Simon, L, Emery, B, & Carrell, DT (2019). Sperm DNA fragmentation: consequences for reproduction. In *Genetic Damage in Human Spermatozoa* (pp. 87-105). Springer, Cham.

[45] Steel AJ, Sutcliffe A. Long-term health implications for children conceived by IVF/ICSI. *Human fertility*. 2009 Jan 1;12(1):21-7.

[46] Tang L, Liu Z, Zhang R, Su C, Yang W, Yao Y, Zhao S. Imprinting alterations in sperm may not significantly influence ART outcomes

and imprinting patterns in the cord blood of offspring. *PloS one.* 2017 Nov 14;12(11):e0187869.

[47] Tsai, PJS, Yamauchi, Y, Riel, JM, & Ward, MA (2020). Pregnancy environment, and not preconception, leads to fetal growth restriction and congenital abnormalities associated with diabetes. *Scientific reports*, *10*(1), 1-11.

[48] Wennerholm UB, Bergh C. Perinatal outcome in children born after assisted reproductive technologies. *Upsala journal of medical sciences.* 2020 Apr 2;125(2):158-66.

[49] Xi, Q, Zhang, Z, Wang, R, Li, L, Li, L, Zhu, H, Liu, R and Luo, L, 2019. Obstetric and perinatal outcomes of intracytoplasmic sperm injection for infertile men with Y chromosome microdeletions. *Medicine*, *98*(41).

[50] Yang M, Fan XB, Wu JN, Wang JM. Association of assisted reproductive technology and multiple pregnancies with the risks of birth defects and stillbirth: A retrospective cohort study. *Scientific reports.* 2018 May 29;8(1):1-8.

[51] Yu Y, Wang R, Xi Q, Zhang H, Jiang Y, Li L, Liu R, Zhang X. Effect of paternal age on intracytoplasmic sperm injection outcomes in cryptozoospermic men: Ejaculated or testicular sperm?. *Medicine.* 2019 Jun;98(26).

[52] Yu Y, Xi Q, Jing J, Li L, Zhang H, Liu R, Pan Y. Intracytoplasmic sperm injection outcome of ejaculated spermatozoa from a man with mosaic Klinefelter's Syndrome: case report and literature review. *Journal of International Medical Research.* 2018 Oct;46(10):4323-31.

[53] Yu Y, Xi Q, Pan Y, Jiang Y, Zhang H, Li L, Liu R. Pregnancy and neonatal outcomes in azoospermic men after intracytoplasmic sperm injection using testicular sperm and donor sperm. *Medical science monitor: international medical journal of experimental and clinical research.* 2018;24:6968.

[54] Zádori J, Kozinszky Z, Orvos H, Katona M, Kaáli SG, Pál A. The incidence of major birth defects following in vitro fertilization. *Journal of assisted reproduction and genetics.* 2003 Mar;20(3): 131-2.

In: Intracytoplasmic Sperm Injection (ICSI) ISBN: 978-1-53619-762-4
Editor: Murid Javed

Chapter 8

Possibility of Transmission of Paternal Genetic Defects through Intracytoplasmic Sperm Injection (ICSI)

Basmah Fraij Alomrani*
Genetics Department, King Abdulaziz University,
Jeddah, Saudi Arabia

Abstract

The current chapter reviews the implementation of ICSI as an assisted reproductive technique in fertilization process in cases of severe male factor infertility, advanced age, and for men who have genetic defects. The literature reviewed showed that there was a high possibility of transmission of paternal genetic defects through ICSI to offspring. The most commonly reported transmitted genetic defects were Klinefelter syndrome to male offspring (47 XXY, 47 XYY genetic defects), severe oligozoospermia, abnormal sperm morphology, fetal hormonal defects, fetal de novo chromosomal abnormalities, and Y chromosomes microdeletions.

* Corresponding Author's E-mail: Basmah.f.alomrani@gmail.com.

Keywords: Genetic defects, oligozoospermia, klienfelter syndrome, Y chromosome microdeletions, hormonal defects, asthenospermia

Introduction

Intracytoplasmic sperm injection (ICSI) is the most commonly utilized fertilization method in assisted reproductive technology worldwide (66.5%; Adamson et al. 2018). It is used exclusively in most of the fertility centers. It is the method of choice for severe male factor infertility, surgically retrieved sperm, for advanced maternal age, low number of oocytes, in vitro matured oocytes, cryopreserved oocytes, and in cases of preimplantation genetic testing (PGT) cases (Adamson et al. 2018).

The utilization of ICSI has increased worldwide. In the Middle-East, its use increased from 58.4% to 98.4%. In the United States, its utilization increased from 36.4% in 1996 to 76.2% in 2012, and reached to 79.29% in 2016, according to the international Committee for Monitoring Assisted Reproductive Technologies (Dyer et al. 2008; Boulet et al. 2015).

Klinefelter Syndrome (47 XXY and 47 XYY Genetic Defects)

The ICSI is used to fertilize eggs by a sperm that is not likely to achieve pregnancy by natural means, and sometimes it must be used for a man carrying a genetic defect. Demily et al. (2017) indicated that Klinefelter syndrome (occurs only in males) 47 XXY or 47 XXXY, Turner syndrome (occurs only in females; 45 X), and 47 XYY syndromes (occurs only in males) are the sex chromosome aneuploidies/disorders which occurred almost one in 420 live births. Klinefelter syndrome (47 XXY) resulted from the presence of one or more X chromosomes in males (**Figure 1C**). Approximately 50% of males with Klinefelter syndrome can produce sperm in a very low concentration. Such men can have their biological offspring through ICSI (Paduch et al. 2008; Plotton et al. 2011; Corona et al. 2017).

Greco et al. (2013) conducted a study to examine the possibility of transmission of paternal chromosomal defects (non-mosaic Klinefelter syndrome, 47 XXY) to offspring. For 26 ICSI cycles performed with ten fresh sperm and sixteen cryopreserved-thawed sperm, the delivery rate was 60% (six out of ten for fresh sperm) and 31.3% (five out of sixteen for frozen-thawed sperm), respectively. It was reported that all offspring were in good health and chromosomally normal (Greco et al. 2013). Zhang et al. (2020) carried out a retrospective study to assess the pregnancy outcomes of paternal sperm with a 47 XYY karyotype utilizing ICSI or in vitro fertilization (IVF).

The study was conducted using data of medical records for 21 patients with a 47 XYY karyotype aged from 21 to 41 years with a mean±SD age of 28.1 ± 5.2 years. Out of 21 patients, three males underwent fertility treatment.

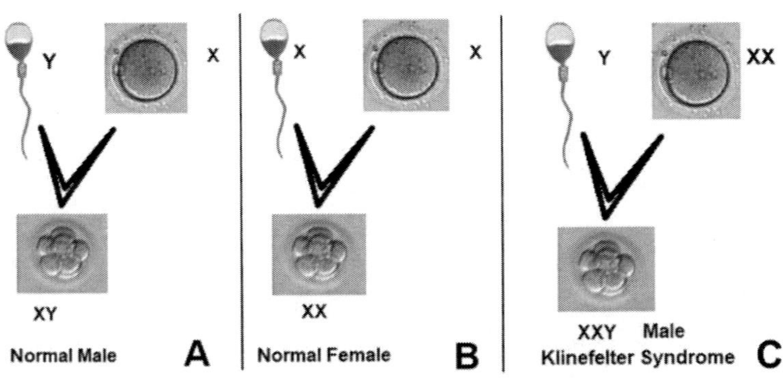

Figure 1. Humans have 46 chromosomes, including two sex chromosomes that determine a person's sex. Females have two X sex chromosomes (XX). Males have an X and a Y sex chromosome (XY). In normal male fertilization, a sperm carrying Y chromosomes fertilizes an oocyte, and the genetic make up of the baby is 46 XY (A). In normal female fertilization a sperm carrying X chromosome fertilizes an egg and the genetic make up of the baby is 46 XX (B). Any variation from 46 XY or 46 XX is considered abnormal genotype. In Klinefelter syndrome, the baby carries 2 X chromosomes and a Y chromosomes and the genetic makeup is 47 XXY (C).

Semen samples were collected after three to five days of sexual abstinence and analyzed based on the fifth edition of the World Health

Organization standard protocol. The patients were diagnosed with oligozoospermia ($<20\times10^6$/mL), moderate oligozoospermia ($>5\times10^6$/mL and $<10\times10^6$/mL), and severe oligozoospermia ($<5\times10^6$/mL) based on the sperm counts of their semen samples. Also, patients were diagnosed with asthenospermia if sperm progressive motility was <50% and with azoospermia if no sperm was present in at least three ejaculates after centrifugation (Zhang et al. 2020). Hormonal, karyotype, and Y chromosome microdeletion analyses were performed, ovarian stimulation was performed according to Liu et al. (2017), ICSI was utilized at 42 hours of human chorionic gonadotropin (hCG) injection and IVF after 40 hours of hCG injection, and embryos were classified based on cleavage rate and morphology score (Zhang et al. 2020).

The study results showed that the incidence of 47 XYY syndrome was 0.1% (21/19,842), a paternal error was reported as the embryo inherits 2 Y chromosomes and semen analysis showed that men with 47 XYY syndrome had sperm count ranged from normal to azoospermia. Abnormal hormonal level, lower testosterone level, and higher FSH and/or LH levels were reported that were considered as indicators of chromosomal defects in those men. The fertilization rate ranged from 52.94% to 83.33%, a boy with normal phenotype was delivered at 38 weeks gestation for patients who used two fresh embryos, while another patients used embryo transfer with frozen-thawed embryos gave birth to a boy with a normal phenotype at 39 weeks gestation, while the third patient didn't have a clinical pregnancy after two frozen-thawed embryos were transferred. Normal karyotype and no deletions on the Y chromosome were reported for those born boys (Zhang et al. 2020).

While, other studies reported that men with XYY syndrome had impaired chromosome synapsis, missed a meiotic recombination site that increases the occurrence of meiotic arrest and increases aneuploidy level within spermatozoa. That means majority of pachytene cells in the patient's ejaculate containing extra Y chromosome ranged from 58% to 100%. All these abnormalities increase the risk of fetal demise and transmission of sex chromosome aneuploidies to the offspring (Ioannou et al. 2015; Wu et al. 2016; Wong et al. 2008; Zhang et al. 2020). Additionally, another study reported that men with XYY syndrome could father children using ART technique (ICSI or IVF) but the risk of transmission of genetic anomalies to offspring is elevated (Enciso et al. 2013).

SEVERE OLIGOZOOSPERMIA OUTCOME

Coates et al. (2015) carried out a retrospective cohort study to compare between the rate of autosome and sex chromosome aneuploidy of embryos derived from sperm with abnormal and normal parameters. Patients were divided into two treatment groups as follows, the 1st group underwent ICSI with normal semen parameters and the second one underwent ICSI, because male patients were with severe oligozoospermia (>19 x 10^6 /mL and <6 x 10^6 /mL sperm, respectively). Another control group of patients who used standard insemination with normal sperm (Table 1) was used to assess the effect of the ICSI technique itself by comparing aneuploidy rate in embryos derived from that control group and ICSI with normal sperm. Six groups were examined for maternal age (own eggs group with mean maternal age of 35.5, 35.3 and 35.3 years and the donor eggs group with mean maternal age of 24.9, 24.9 and 25.0, respectively). Kruskal–Wallis one-way analysis of variance on ranks was used to assess the differences in aneuploidy rates for each chromosome pair. The second group of male patients with severe oligozoospermia showed a significant higher chromosome aneuploidy reaching to threefold than the other two groups using either donor or own eggs. Additionally, oligozoospermic group showed a significant difference for autosomes 1, 2, 13 for own eggs (older), and 18 for donor eggs (younger), compared to the other two groups. No significant variation was reported between all treatment groups regarding the overall rate of autosomal aneuploidy and the two treatment control groups (standard or ICSI with normal sperm) in terms of the type of the egg group for any chromosome pairs. Therefore, the authors concluded that a significant association was found between the increase in occurrence of sex chromosome abnormalities in blastocyst embryos and severe male infertility (oligozoospermia), compared with the embryo derived from normal semen samples. Also, there was no significant difference regarding the rate of aneuploidy in embryos derived from sperm with normal parameters whether ICSI or standard insemination procedure were used for fertilization, so the study indicated that the risk of chromosomal abnormalities occurrence is associated with infertile father with low quality of spermatozoa rather than the ICSI technique itself (Coates et al. 2015).

Therefore, the study shed the light on the necessity of comprehensive chromosomal screening (American Society for Reproductive Medicine 2015). These results agreed with Gabriel et al. (2011) and Wen et al. (2012).

ABNORMAL EMBRYO MORPHOLOGY

Ramasamy et al. (2015) conducted a study and showed that paternal semen with poor sperm morphology is more likely to have a high incidence of autosomal aneuploidy in their sperm and a higher rate of sperm aneuploidy for chromosomes 13, 18, and 21.

Table 1. Lower reference limits (5th centiles and their 95% confidence intervals) for semen characteristics

Parameter	Reference Value
Semen volume (ml)	1.5 (1.4–1.7)
Sperm concentration (10^6 per ml)	15 (12–16)
Total motility (PR + NP, %)	40 (38–42)
Progressive motility (PR, %)	32 (31–34)
Sperm morphology (normal forms, %)	4 (3.0–4.0)

Adopted from *WHO laboratory manual for the examination and processing of human semen*, 5th Ed. (2010), Appendix 1. World Health Organization.

Also, two studies reported that increase in the risk of congenital abnormalities is associated with paternal subfertility not to ICSI as a fertilization method (Wen et al. 2012; Hansen et al. 2013).

Mendoza et al. (2015) conducted a retrospective case-control study to examine the association between very poor-quality embryo (congenital malformations and chromosomal abnormalities) and paternal problems through undergoing IVF or ICSI. In total 74 children derived from IVF and/or ICSI resulting from the transfer of very poor-quality embryo were compared with 1,507 children delivered after the transfer of top morphological quality embryos whose are considered the control group, during the same period in the same reproductive centers. It was reported that the prevalence of birth defects was similar in children who are delivered from very poor-quality embryos and from top quality morphology (1.35% and 1.72%, respectively). Additionally, the rate of chromosomal abnormalities was similar, there was no case of perinatal mortality in the group of very-poor quality embryo (0%), while the group of very good morphology embryo had 20 cases of perinatal mortality (13%), among them only in one case the death was due to congenital malformations. It was concluded that the rate of perinatal complications and congenital malformations didn't seem to be more common/higher in patients after transfer of very poor quality embryos through IVF and/or ICSI procedures. The authors added that if no other embryos are available, the transfer of a poor-quality embryo shouldn't be excluded to avoid perinatal complications or congenital malformations in the offspring (Hansen et al. 2013).

Fetal Hormonal Defects

Belva et al. (2016) conducted a longitudinal cohort study and reported that boys delivered through ICSI had a significant increase in LH: testosterone ratio and reduction in free and total serum testosterone levels, compared to naturally conceived boys. However, there was no difference in hormonal profile of boys conceived with IVF or natural conception. Also, there was no difference between boys conceived with ICSI or IVF regarding serum reproductive hormone concentrations. Therefore, the authors demonstrated that the impairment in Leydig cell function in boys conceived through ICSI is possibly inherited from their fathers who had impaired Leydig cell function and decreased serum testosterone level. These results are supported by other studies by Belva et al. (2017) and Belva et al. (2020).

De-Novo Chromosomal Abnormalities

Belva et al. (2020) carried out a study to assess the association between ICSI and paternal semen parameters using fetal karyotype abnormalities. Results of postnatal blood sample from offspring conceived by ICSI and results from prenatal testing (amniocentesis and chorionic villus sampling) were taken to report karyotype results. Also, pregnancies that resulted from oocyte retrieval and post transfer of fresh ICSI embryos using fresh ejaculated or frozen-thawed sperm were taken into consideration. The cases using preimplantation genetic testing, IVF, IVM, frozen embryo transfer, and sperm or oocyte donation were excluded. All abnormal prenatal results were reported regardless of the pregnancy outcome. Out of 4816 ICSI pregnancies only 4267 pregnancies outcome data were available. The prenatal tests were utilized in 22.3% of the pregnancies while a postnatal karyotype was obtained in 29.4% of all pregnancies in which prenatal diagnosis was not performed. The prevalence of chromosomal anomalies was analyzed according to maternal age and semen quality. The study results showed that 29 singletons and 12 multiples had an abnormal fetal karyotype, among them 36 anomalies were de novo [numerical (n = 25), sex (n = 6), or structural (n = 5), and five are inherited] (41/1114; 3.7%; 95% CI 2.7 – 4.9%, 3.2%; 95% CI 2.3 - 4.4, respectively). There was no significant association between a de novo chromosomal fetal abnormality and mother's age. Out of 1391 postnatal samples of newborn after ICSI, 14 had abnormal karyotypes that didn't undergo prenatal testing and born after ICSI using ejaculated sperm, only two of them inherited balanced karyotype and twelve were de novo anomalies. Increasing maternal age increased the risk of karyotype aberration as shown by comparing between prenatal and postnatal data. Fetuses with an abnormal karyotype were conceived by ICSI using ejaculated sperm. The fetuses of men with a sperm concentration of <5 million/ml showed a higher rate of de novo chromosomal abnormalities (Belva et al. 2020).

Therefore, the same study concluded that ICSI offspring with a higher rate of de novo chromosomal abnormalities in prenatal and postnatal karyotypes are associated with paternal sperm parameters (having sperm concentration below reference sperm concentrations) (Belva et al. 2020).

Y CHROMOSOME MICRODELETIONS

Hu et al. (2019) published a case-report study of a 27-year old man with Y-chromosome microdeletions and 2 year of primary infertility. Semen analysis based on World Health Organization guidelines showed normal fresh semen volume and severe oligoasthenospermia, where the concentration was 0.27million/mL, the motility of sperm was rare on microscopic examination. The karyotype analysis of the patients was 46, XY, inv (9) (p11q13), while karyotype analysis of his wife was normal. According to PCR analysis, two markers were deleted (sY254 and sY255) and other STS markers were found for AZFa (sY84 and sY86) and for AZFb (sY127, sY134, and sY143) that means absence of deletions in these regions (AZFc microdeletions). The patient underwent ICSI procedure, out of 9 oocytes collected, only two fertilized. Two embryos were transferred to the patient's wife uterus on day 3. After two weeks of embryo transfer, the serum concentration of βhCG was 256.3 mIU/ml confirming pregnancy. After 39 weeks of gestations, a healthy girl was born, and the pregnancy was at high risk for trisomy 21 syndrome (risk value: 1 in 150) through the results of second-trimester maternal serum triple-screening. From cultured amniocytes, the karyotype of the fetus was 46 XX, inv (9) (p11q13). It was concluded that an abnormal karyotype (inv (9) (p11q13) of paternal with Y-chromosome AZFc microdeletions was transmitted to his offspring through ICSI (Hu Cong et al., 2019). While Bonne et al. (2016) reported that prenatal screening serum markers' values can be affected by ICSI and/or IVF when screening for trisomy 21.

García-Peiró et al. (2011) reported that men with infertility and inv (9) karyotype had significant anomalous aneuploidy, meiotic alterations, high levels of sperm DNA fragmentation, and altered seminogram parameters, which resulted in chromosomal imbalance in offspring.

Conclusion

Examination of paternal karyotype for men undergoing ICSI and genetic counseling are recommended for men especially with severe oligozoospermia. The evidence indicates that paternal chromosomal anomalies can be transmitted through ICSI technique as severely oligozoospermic or asthenospermic sample is not likely to result in natural conception. Therefore, the men desiring to have a biological child should be made aware of this fact. The ICSI technique itself is not causing chromosomal defects. The preimplantation genetic testing and transfer of euploid embryo (s) is recommended in cases with abnormal parental Karyotype.

References

[1] Adamson, G., de Mouzon, J., Chambers, G., Zegers-Hochschild, F., Mansour, R., Ishihara, O. et al. International Committee for Monitoring Assisted Reproductive Technology: World report on assisted reproductive technology, 2011. *Fertil. Steril.,* 2018; 110(06): 1067 - 79.

[2] American Society for Reproductive Medicine, *Fertil. Steril.,* 2015; 104(4): 866 - 72.

[3] Belva, F., Bonduelle, M., Buysse, A., Van den, A., Bogaert, F., Hes, M., Roelants, G., Verheyen, H. et al. Chromosomal abnormalities after ICSI in relation to semen parameters: results in 1114 fetuses and 1391 neonates from a single center, *Human Reproduction*, 2020;35: 2149 - 2162.

[4] Belva, F. Semen quality of young adult ICSI offspring: The first results. *Hum. Reprod.,* 2016; 31:2811 - 2820.

[5] Belva, F. Serum reproductive hormone levels and ultrasound findings in female offspring after intracytoplasmic sperm injection: First results. *Fertil. Steril.,* 2017; 107:934 - 939.

[6] Bonne, S., Sauleau, E., Sananes, N. et al. Influence of medically assisted reproduction techniques on crown-rump length and

biochemical markers of trisomy 21 in the first trimester of pregnancy. *Fertil. Steril.,* 2016; 105:410 - 6.

[7] Boulet, S. L., Mehta, A., Kissin, D. M., Warner, L., Kawwass, J. F., Jamieson, D. J. Trends in use of and reproductive outcomes associated with intracytoplasmic sperm injection. *JAMA,* 2015; 313: 255 - 263. (10.1001/jama.2014.17985).

[8] Coates, A., Hesla, J. S., Hurliman, A., Coate, B., Holmes, E., Matthews, R., Mounts, E. L., Turner, K. J., Thornhill, A. R., Griffin, D. K. Use of suboptimal sperm increases the risk of aneuploidy of the sex chromosomes in preimplantation blastocyst embryos. *Fertil. Steril.,* 2015; 104(4):866 - 872. doi: 10.1016/j.fertnstert.2015.06.033.

[9] Corona, G., Pizzocaro, A., Lanfranco, F., Garolla, A., Pelliccione, F., Vignozzi, L., Ferlin, A., Foresta, C., Jannini, E. A., Maggi, M., Lenzi, A., Pasquali, D., Francavilla, S. Klinefelter ItaliaN Group (KING). Sperm recovery and ICSI outcomes in Klinefelter syndrome: A systematic review and meta-analysis. *Hum. Reprod. Update*, 2017 May 1; 23(3):265 - 275. doi: 10.1093/humupd/dmx008.

[10] Demily, C., Poisson, A., Peyroux, E. et al. Autism spectrum disorder associated with 49, XYYYY: Case report and review of the literature. *BMC Med. Genet.,* 2017; 18:9.

[11] Dyer, S., Chambers, G. M., de Mouzon, J., Nygren, K. G., Zegers-Hochschild, F., Mansour, R., Ishihara, O., Banker, M., Adamson, G. D. International Committee for Monitoring Assisted Reproductive Technologies world report: Assisted Reproductive Technology 2008, 2009 and 2010. *Human Reproduction*, 2016; 31:1588 - 1609.

[12] Enciso, M., Alfarawati, S., Wells, D. Increased numbers of DNA-damaged spermatozoa in samples presenting an elevated rate of numerical chromosome abnormalities. *Hum. Reprod.,* 2013; 28:1707 - 15.

[13] Gabriel, A. S., Hassold, T. J., Thornhill, A. R., Affara, N. A., Handyside, A. H., Griffin, D. K. An algorithm for determining the origin of trisomy and the positions of chiasmata from SNP genotype data. *Chromosome Res.,* 2011; 19:155 - 63.

[14] García-Peiró, A., Oliver-Bonet, M., Navarro, J. et al. Dynamics of sperm DNA fragmentation in patients carrying structurally rearranged chromosomes. *Int. J. Androl.,* 2011; 34:e546 - 53.

[15] Greco, E., Scarselli, F., Minasi, M. G., Casciani, V., Zavaglia, D., Dente, D., Tesarik, J., Franco, G. Birth of 16 healthy children after ICSI in cases of nonmosaic Klinefelter syndrome. *Hum. Reprod.,* 2013 May; 28(5):1155 - 60. doi: 10.1093/humrep/det046.

[16] Hansen, M., Kurinczuk, J. J., Milne, E., de Klerk, N., Bower, C. Assisted reproductive technology and birth defects: A systematic review and meta- analysis. *Hum. Reprod. Update*, 2013; 19:330 - 353.

[17] Hu Cong, M. M., Xiangy, L., Linlin, L., Xiaonan, H., Haibo, Z., Dongfeng, G. et al. The reproductive outcome of an infertile man with AZFc microdeletions, via intracytoplasmic sperm injection in a high-risk pregnancy, *Medicine,* 2019; 98:16358 doi: 10.1097/ MD.0000000000016358.

[18] Ioannou, D., Tempest, H. G. Meiotic nondisjunction: insights into the origin and significance of aneuploidy in human spermatozoa. *Adv. Exp. Med. Biol.,* 2015; 868:1 - 21.

[19] Liu, X. Y., Wang, R. X., Fu, Y. Outcomes of intracytoplasmic sperm injection in oligozoospermic men with Y chromosome AZFb or AZFc microdeletions. *Andrologia,* 2017; 49:12602.

[20] Mendoza, R., Perez, S., de Los Santos, M. J., Larreategui, Z., Ayerdi, F., Expósito, A., Burgos, J., Martínez Indart, L., Pijoan, J. I., Matorras, R. Congenital malformations, chromosomal abnormalities and perinatal results in IVF/ICSI newborns resulting from very poor quality embryos: A case-control study. *Gynecol. Obstet. Invest.,* 2015; 79(2): 83 - 9. doi: 10.1159/000353605.

[21] Paduch, D. A., Fine, R. G., Bolyakov, A., Kiper, J. New concepts in Klinefelter syndrome. *Current Opinion in Urology,* 2008. Nov. 1; 18(6):621 - 7.

[22] Palermo, G. D., Neri, Q. V., Rosenwaks, Z. 2015b. To ICSI or Not to ICSI. *Seminars in Reproductive Medicine*, 2015b; 33:92 - 102. (10.1055/s-0035-1546825).

[23] Plotton, I., Brosse, A., Lejeune, H. Infertility treatment in Klinefelter syndrome. Gynecologie, *Obstetrique and Fertilite,* 2011. Aug. 10; 39(9):529 - 32.

[24] Ramasamy, R., Scovell, J. M., Kovac, J. R., Cook, P. J., Lamb, D. J., Lipshultz, L. I. Fluorescence in situ hybridization detects increased sperm aneuploidy in men with recurrent pregnancy loss. *Fertil. Steril.,* 2015; 103:906 - 9.

[25] Wen, J., Jiang, J., Ding, C., Dai, J., Liu, Y., Xia, Y. Birth defects in children conceived by in vitro fertilization and intracytoplasmic sperm injection: A meta-analysis. *Fertil. Steril.,* 2012; 97:1331 - 7.

[26] Wong, E. C., Ferguson, K. A., Chow, V. Sperm aneuploidy and meiotic sex chromosome configurations in an infertile XYY male. *Hum. Reprod.*, 2008; 23:374 - 8.

[27] Wu, C., Wang, L., Iqbal, F. Preferential Y-Y pairing and synapsis and, abnormal meiotic recombination in a 47, XYY man with non obstructive azoospermia. *Mol. Cytogenetic,* 2016; 9:9.

[28] *WHO laboratory manual for the examination and processing of human semen*, 5th Ed (2010), Appendix 1. World Health Organization. Pp. 224.

[29] Zhang, X., Liu, X., Xi, Q. Reproductive outcomes of 3 infertile males with XYY syndrome: Retrospective case series and literature review. *Medicine,* (Baltimore). 2020; 99(9):e19375. doi:10.1097/ MD.0000000000019375.

EDITOR CONTACT INFORMATION

Murid Javed, PhD
Laboratory Director
OriginElle Fertility Clinic and Women's Health Centre,
Ottawa and Montreal, Canada
E-mail: murid.javed@gmail.com

INDEX

#

A

B

C

D

N

O

P

Q

R

S

T

U

V

W

X

Y

Z